Embracing the Journey

Moving Forward After Brain Injury

Embracing the Journey

Moving Forward After Brain Injury

by Amy Zellmer
A collection of short stories originally
published on *HuffPost*

Embracing the Journey
Moving Forward After Brain Injury
©Copyright 2018 by Amy Zellmer
All rights reserved.

22 21 20 19 18   5 4 3 2 1

ISBN: 9781985320192

Library of Congress: 2018901216

First Printing 2018

Published by Amy Zellmer, Saint Paul, Minnesota
Edited by Connie Anderson, Words & Deeds, Inc.
Cover photo and design by Amy Zellmer
Interior Design by FuzionPrint.com
Interior photos property of Amy Zellmer

Embracing the Journey Moving Forward After Brain Injury is a work of nonfiction. The names, details, and circumstances may have been changed to protect the survivor's identity.

Dedicated to my Tribe

Table of Contents

Chapter	Title	Page
Chapter 1	It's Not Just A Concussion	21
Chapter 2	Healing From Traumatic Brain Injury With Yoga	27
Chapter 3	"You Look Great"—Life With a TBI	33
Chapter 4	Quit Using Your Brain Injury As An Excuse	39
Chapter 5	Four Lessons I Learned From NASCAR About Concussions	45
Chapter 6	Ben Utecht, NFL Champ, Writes Book About Concussions And Memory Loss	49
Chapter 7	Let's Talk About Sex...After Brain Injury	55
Chapter 8	Five Symptoms of PTSD After Brain Injury	63
Chapter 9	How Functional Neurology Helped Improve My Quality of Life After Brain Injury	71
Chapter 10	Eye Movements May Be Key In Detecting Brain Injury, Concussion	81
Chapter 11	A Struggle Back to Financial Freedom After a Brain Injury	89

Chapter 12   Who Rescued Whom? How My   **97**
              Yorkie Helped Me Cope After Brain
              Injury

Chapter 13   The Many Personalities of Brain   **101**
              Injury—Why I Sometimes Want to
              Throw in the Towel

Chapter 14   Understanding Aphasia After Brain   **107**
              Injury

Chapter 15   Living in a Funk: Depression and   **113**
              Apathy After Brain Injury

Chapter 16   Pediatric Hospital Creates Abilities **119**
              Adventures Program For Brain
              Injury Patients

Chapter 17   The Downside of Functional   **125**
              Neurology After Brain Injury

Chapter 18   Six Tips for Surviving the Holidays **133**
              and Overstimulation With a TBI

Chapter 19   It's Not Like You Have Cancer or   **139**
              Something

Chapter 20   Former Wall Street Exec Turns   **145**
              Focus to Concussion and Brain
              Health

Chapter 21   How Minnesota Is Helping to Solve   **153**
              the Concussion Epidemic Through
              Research and Innovation

Chapter 22   Spotlights: Brain Injury Advisory   **167**
              Council Members

Chapter 23   An Open Letter to Arianna   **183**
              Huffington

Statistics

All information in this section is cited and shared with permission from the Centers for Disease Control and Prevention (CDC).

Overview

Traumatic brain injury (TBI) is a major cause of death and disability in the United States, contributing to about 30 percent of all injury-related deaths. Every day, 153 people in the United States die from injuries that include TBI. Those who survive a TBI can face effects lasting a few days—to disabilities that may last the rest of their lives. Effects of TBI can include impaired thinking or memory, movement, sensation (e.g., vision or hearing), or emotional function (e.g., personality changes, depression). These issues not only affect the individual, but can have lasting effects on families and communities.

What is a TBI?

A TBI is caused by a bump, blow, or jolt to the head, or a penetrating head injury that disrupts the normal function of the brain. Not all blows or jolts to the head result in a TBI. The severity of a TBI may range from "mild" to "severe." Most TBIs that occur each year are mild, commonly called concussions. Doctors may describe a concussion as a "mild" brain injury because concussions are usually not life-threatening. Even so, their effects can be serious.

Statistics

- Every 11 seconds someone in the United States will suffer a TBI.
- Each year a reported 2.8 million people will sustain a TBI.
- TBI contributes to the deaths of nearly 55,000 people each year.
- The number of unreported TBIs, or those not seen by a doctor, is unknown.
- In 2013, falls were the leading cause of TBIs. Falls accounted for 47 percent of all TBI-related emergency room visits, hospitalizations, and deaths in the United States. Falls disproportionately affect the youngest and the oldest age groups.
- More than half (54%) of TBI-related ED (emergency department) visits, hospitalizations, and deaths among children 0 to 14.
- Nearly 4 in 5 (79%) TBI-related ED visits, hospitalizations, and deaths in adults aged 65 and older.
- Being struck by or against an object was the second leading cause of TBI, accounting for about 15 percent of TBI-related ED visits, hospital-izations, and deaths in the United States in 2013.

- More than 1 in 5 (22%) TBI-related ED visits, hospitalizations, and deaths in children less than 15 years of age.
- Among all age groups, motor vehicle crashes were the third overall leading cause of TBI-relations ED visits, hospitalizations, and deaths (14%). When looking at only TBI-related deaths, motor vehicle crashes were also the third leading cause (19%) in 2013.
- Intentional self-harm was the second leading cause of TBI-related deaths (33%) in 2013.

Foreword

Brain injury does not discriminate. Anytime, anywhere, anyone can acquire a brain injury from trauma, stroke, sports, or drug overdose that can change the way you walk, talk, think, and feel. In fact, more than 2.8 million people in the United States sustain brain injuries each year.

Recovery from brain injury is not easy. Stingy health insurance plans limit the amount of rehabilitation that patients can access, and gaping holes in America's social safety net put the burden of lifelong care on individual survivors and their families.

Few people are equipped to handle brain injury alone. Fortunately, they don't have to!

The Brain Injury Association of America is the nation's oldest and largest brain injury advocacy organization. With a network of state affiliates, the Association provides information and resources through a toll-free National Brain Injury Information Center at 1-800-444-6443 and online at www.biausa.org.

For nearly 40 years, people with brain injury and their caregivers have been telling their stories, to both heal themselves and inspire others. Every story is different because the wisdom gained from each experience is different. Plus, each person brings his or her own style and personality to the tale. The tips, tricks, and lessons learned in living with brain injury help others recover, accept themselves, and adapt to a new life.

This collection of essays by Amy Zellmer, a master storyteller, shows what persistence, determination, and acceptance can achieve—even when there's no clear understanding of what life might bring next. Amy's stories are both honest and inspiring. They put the reality of brain injury on display, showing the challenges, victories, and setbacks that millions of Americans face each day. Importantly, Amy's stories illustrate the impact individuals with brain injury can have in raising awareness among opinion leaders and policymakers.

Enjoy.

Susan H. Connors, President/CEO
Brain Injury Association of America

Acknowledgments

This book was a labor of love, and many people helped me on this journey.

I wish to thank these people:

Toni, for being my biggest cheerleader (and supplying me with Nutella snacks).

Simon, for making sure I always had enough sushi to eat, and a shoulder to lean on.

The Women of Words ladies, for tremendous encouragement, love and support.

My fellow advocates locally and nationally; together we are creating awareness and giving voice to TBI.

Jeff and Erica, for helping to shape me into the advocate that I am today.

Toni, Paul, Stephanie, Anne, and Amy, for being the greatest friends and survivors I could ask for.

Dr. Schmoe, for without your compassion and understanding of TBI, I wouldn't be where I am in my recovery today.

I would like to thank my Kickstarter backers who pledged at the "recognition" reward level

Christine Fitch

Cindy Nester

Cognitive FX

Cyn Ladd

Jami Benz

Jennifer Malocha

Julie Castell

Justin Sinks

A HUGE thank you to every single backer from $1 to $500...you all helped make this book possible.

Introduction

When I first fell in February 2014, I never imagined the incredible journey that a TBI would take me on. I have turned my focus away from professional photography, which has been my career path the past 20 years, and towards advocacy and awareness. In the years after I first fell, I felt isolated, alone, and scared. I didn't know if I was ever going to get better, or find my way back to normal. Since writing my first book, *Life With a Traumatic Brain Injury: Finding the Road Back to Normal,* I have found the right doctors, and have a renewed sense of hope. This book starts up where the first one ended.

I realized that when I finally embraced who I was, and that my writing could instill hope and inspiration in others who were on a similar journey, I was able to allow myself the ability to heal. It wasn't until I told myself: "Amy—put on your big-girl panties! This might be the best you're going to get, and that's OK!"

Finding Dr. Schmoe was a profound turn of events for my recovery. Well, actually he found me, through one of my *HuffPost* articles. Working with a Functional Neurologist who is specially trained in treating concussion and brain injury was life changing—literally.

I continued to write, and as a result I would hear from hundreds of survivors who resonated with my words. The stories I receive from others are what propel me to continue writing. With the recent very sudden news of *HuffPost* letting go of all their contributors, I am certain that new doors will open for me, and my words will continue to inspire.

My hope is that my writing can help other survivors know they're not alone, help loved ones understand what their survivor is going through, and help healthcare professionals have a glimpse into the life of what their patients are dealing with.

Writing is my therapy, and writing is also my platform to help others around the world.

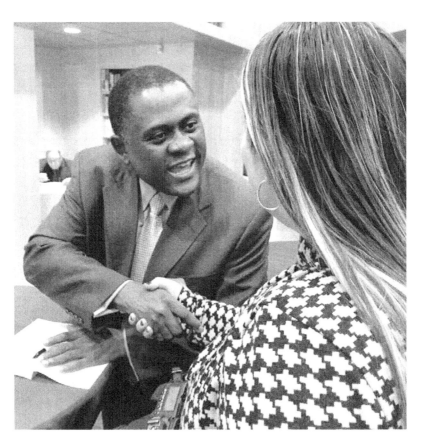

Meeting Dr. Bennett Omalu at a book signing in Minnesota.

Chapter One

It's Not *Just* A Concussion

January 2016

In a society where the result of a severe bump on the head is often overlooked, misdiagnosed, and misunderstood, the word "concussion" should *not* be taken lightly. Every concussion is a traumatic brain injury and needs to be taken seriously—*as it is the leading cause of death for children and adults ages 1–44 in the United States—and occurs every 11 seconds.*

With the 2015 movie "Concussion" starring Will Smith, we are finally starting to talk about it. While the movie is about NFL players and their concussions, I understood every word—every nuance of how these guys felt. I understood their frustration when nobody would listen to them, or take them seriously when their MRIs came back clear.

You don't have to be in a serious car accident or injured playing sports. Simply slipping on a patch of ice can change your life in the blink of an eye, which is exactly what happened to me.

It was a very cold February morning when I slipped and fell on a patch of sheer ice while walking down my building's driveway. I remember my feet flying out from under me, in true Charlie Brown fashion, and I was unable to do anything about it. I can still hear the god-awful "thunk" as my head made contact with the asphalt. *My skull had taken the full impact of the fall,* knocking me unconscious for a few minutes.

When I came to, I immediately knew something was wrong. The pain in my skull was excruciating, and I was seeing whirly stars out of my left eye. Once back in the safety of my apartment, I attempted to look up emergency rooms on Google. Then I realized I couldn't read my computer screen—it was a blur because my eyes wouldn't focus. Calling 911 hadn't even occurred to me. Because I had clearly knocked myself silly, I decided I would drive to the clinic. A decision I look back on and realize it probably wasn't a good one.

After a thorough exam, my doctor told me I had suffered a severe concussion, along with major whiplash, C4/5 damage to my spine, and a dislocated sternum. He stated my concussion symptoms should start getting better in about six to eight weeks. Before releasing me to go home, I was instructed to cancel all of my appointments for the week, and to avoid all stimulation, including TV, radio, reading, etc. I was to return to the doctor later that evening to ensure I was still doing okay—you know, not dying from a brain bleed or anything.

As weeks, then months, went on, I was still not feeling any better, and in fact, my symptoms were becoming worse. I was living with a constant fogginess in my head, a perpetual headache, and my short-term memory was practically non-existent. And at times I could not find my way home from the neighborhood store or my best friend's house, or remember how to run my microwave. I had trouble finding words when I spoke, I was suffering from dizziness and balance issues, and my vision wasn't quite right, even though eye exams showed everything was "fine."

While I was living with this hell inside my head, friends started to drift away, telling me I should "get over it" because it was 'just' a concussion." One former friend even said I should be thankful it's "just a concussion," and not something far worse, like cancer.

I would eventually come to understand a term I had never heard before: "traumatic brain injury" or TBI for short. *Every concussion is a TBI,* yet when people hear about TBI, they tend to think of the worst-case scenarios. Because I looked seemingly fine, and could walk and talk, people thought I must be okay. I think some people even went so far as to assume I was faking or exaggerating; yet if they had spent even an hour with me, they would realize I wasn't the same person I was before my fall.

The stigma of a concussion in our society is that it is "no big deal." We watch professional athletes get back in the game after taking a major blow to the head, and we expect the same of our youth. We watch actors like Tracy Morgan, who suffered a major TBI after an awful accident involving his tour bus and a semi-truck, tell us a year later that he's 100 percent recovered...while I am grateful to hear he's doing so well, I don't buy the "100 percent recovered" part one bit.

In the movie "Concussion," we start to garner an understanding that concussions are much more serious than originally thought. We get a glimpse inside the severity of repetitive head trauma, and how it can hide invisibly inside our brains, while wreaking havoc on our lives.

My accident was February of 2014, and I am still not completely recovered. I have accepted the reality that I may never be 100 percent the same as I was before, and have adopted coping mechanisms to help me with my short-term memory loss and aphasia (the inability to come up with words, or saying the wrong word). I continue to deal with neuro-fatigue and occasional confusion.

Parents, go see the movie "Concussion," and if your son or daughter takes a physical hit in sports or other activities, monitor them closely, and then don't allow your children back in the game until they have been cleared by a medical professional. Continue to watch your children at home, and if they don't seem like themselves, or are exhibiting other unusual symptoms, take them in for reevaluation, and don't let them continue to play until you're certain they are 100 percent okay.

We must realize children also hit their heads riding a bike or playing on the playground, and with little ones, starting at age one, hitting glass doors and walls as they begin to learn how to walk. We can't keep them and ourselves in a perpetual safety bubble, but we do need to be aware of signs and symptoms. As we learn in the movie, repetitive hits to the head can cause very serious long-term, invisible issues.

Now, instead of hearing "it's 'just' a concussion," I hear *"you look great; you must be recovered."* That's a whole other story for another day. Until you suffer a life-altering brain injury, you will never be able to understand what the other person is going through. I know I sure didn't. It is a long, lonely road to recovery.

When I think back to when I was first going through this, I still shake my head at the ignorance of some people. Actually, I have since learned most people have no idea of the complexities of a TBI. My hope is to help raise awareness about traumatic brain injury, and how serious a concussion really is.

We only get one brain—it's our job to protect it!!

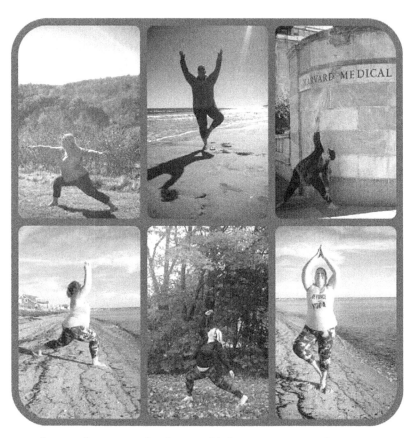

I have photographed myself doing yoga in almost 40 states as part of my accountability project.

Chapter Two

Healing From Traumatic Brain Injury With Yoga

May 2016

Yoga is something I have done since college (if you promise not to do math, I'll simply say I've been doing yoga for twenty-plus years).

There was a period of time when I considered going through the teacher training program and becoming a yoga instructor, and now I really wish I had followed through on that thought.

Why, you ask?

You don't understand yoga's true, full potential until you've gone through a life-changing physical trauma. Knowing what I know now, I have a deeper love and appreciation for yoga, and a greater understanding of its powerful healing benefits.

When I slipped on that patch of black ice on an inclined driveway, I had zero warning as my feet went up into the air and *my skull made full impact with the frozen asphalt.* Amazingly, I walked away with my life. I am still in awe at the incredible resilience of one's skull, and how much of an impact it can actually take.

What I did sustain in the fall included: a severe concussion (later referred to as a traumatic brain injury, or TBI for short), major whiplash, C4/5 damage in my neck, torn muscles in my neck, throat, abdomen, and chest, and a dislocated sternum.

Sounds like a load of fun, huh?

As we began addressing the physical injuries, I was unaware of the journey I was starting inside my head. *A traumatic brain injury is an extremely complicated and invisible injury, and one that many professionals (as well as friends and family) just don't quite understand.* I was frustrated when doctors wouldn't listen to me, or would simply tell me I would feel better in a few weeks. Every few weeks would start a new cycle of pain, grief, and anxiety.

After about 15 months of feeling pained, isolated, depressed, and anxious, I reached out to a yoga instructor friend of mine.

Because of the dislocated sternum, I couldn't lift my hands much higher than my shoulder, nor could I take a full, deep breath. Because of the TBI, I suffered from dizziness, poor balance, and neck mobility issues. I also noticed I would drag my right foot, and my right arm did not move in motion with my walk—both of which are a neurological problem.

My dear friend helped me come up with *five yoga poses* I could do without feeling like I would fall over, or would cause me pain and discomfort.

Five poses. That was it.

They included: cat-cow pose, puppy dog (child's) pose, tree pose (with the help of a chair for balance), eagle arm pose, and side twists while lying down.

After a few days of doing these five poses for about 10 to 15 minutes, *I started noticing a difference.* I was able to breathe deeper than I had since the accident, my flexibility was slowly coming back, and my dizziness and balance issues were starting to bother me less. My range of motion was growing every single time I did yoga.

When I felt ready, I gradually added some of my favorite poses for a single breath. I would go into down-dog pose and warrior pose simply to see if I could. I would hold it for one breath, and then two. I eventually got brave enough to try side angle pose, which is my ultimate favorite pose. I was thrilled that I was able to do it, at least with a block to assist me.

Now as I write this, it's slightly over two years out from my accident, and I am an advocate for TBI awareness. Not only do I want to raise awareness, I want to help other survivors, which brings me back to my point about teacher training. While you do not need an actual license/certificate to teach yoga, *I would very much love to take a course on trauma yoga,* and help other survivors find some comfort and peace in yoga, the way I did.

Everyone can do yoga, even those who think they have to be "flexible" to do it. Yoga is an individual activity, one in which you do only what you can. It can be modified to fit your injury, and some poses can even be done from a hospital bed. *There are amazing benefits to doing yoga, and I hope my experience can help another survivor decide to give it a try*—and do it under the guidance of an instructor.

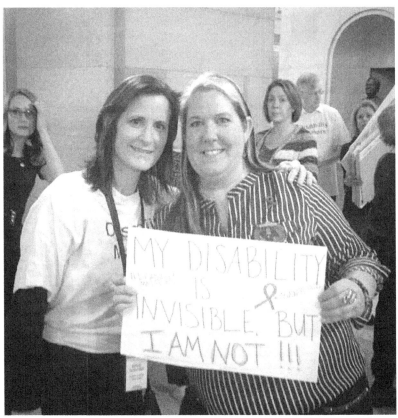

With Erica from the Minnesota Brain Injury Alliance at the Disability Matters Rally at the Minnesota State Capitol.

Chapter Three

"You Look Great"—Life With a TBI

July 2016

"You look great! You must be fully recovered!"
"You look great! You must be feeling good!"
I have come to loathe these phrases. I know they
are usually said with good intentions; however, most often
they are so far from the actual truth it is frustrating to hear.

It's exhausting to give the correct answer, so most of the
time I simply reply, "Thanks, I'm still recovering," to which
I get strange sideways glances. It's as if the fact I am
walking and talking means I can't possibly *still be
recovering* from a traumatic brain injury (TBI).

Invisible injuries are often dismissed by those who don't
truly understand. If we're seen smiling and laughing,
people deem we are fine, yet there is a hell inside our heads
holding us back from actually being able to enjoy whatever
it is we are doing. It takes every ounce of energy I have left
to put on that smile and laugh, all while hoping a headache
doesn't completely take me out before it's an acceptable
time for me to leave.

Once my physical injuries healed, which were also
invisible, I was able to be a bit more active in my daily life,
although I still suffered from intense fatigue, headaches,

brain fog, balance issues, short-term memory loss, aphasia, and vision problems.

> *Casey from Kentucky stated, "Living with any invisible injury is difficult, but when that injury affects the organ that controls your entire body, it is almost impossible for others to understand. Emotions, pain, energy, vision, and even the ability to think clearly have become a daily struggle. Hearing 'you look fine' has become the norm. Time can sometimes heal, but often it just allows those around you to forget."*

Because no one can see inside my brain, I realize it is hard for someone outside of the TBI community to conceptualize what I am going through. But *instead of making assumptions of how I am doing,* based on the fact that I am out and about, ask me *how I am doing.* "How are you feeling today?" or "How is the recovery going?" would be appreciated. I may answer with a simple, "Oh, pretty good," even though I am feeling miserable, but I am thankful you understand I am still recovering, even two-plus years later.

In the beginning, I was very sad that so many friends I thought would be there for me, were slowly disappearing from my life.

I don't know if they thought I was faking, seeking attention, exaggerating, or what. It hurt me in profound ways, yet, I am thankful for them. Their attitudes toward me are what originally provoked me to write about my journey, which ultimately led me to finding my "Tribe" and a whole new circle of friends and people who care deeply about me.

I commonly hear survivors talk about *loss of friend-ships as one of the side effects of TBI.* Outsiders simply don't understand what we are going through, and that leaves us feeling hurt, isolated, and exceedingly alone. Not everyone has a caregiver or someone close by to help that person get through this debilitating injury.

Jan from Arizona has been a caregiver to her partner, Stacy, for the past 15 years after a horrific and bizarre head-on horse-racing incident. She commented, "We have lost the majority of our friends in the past 15 years since Stacy's traumatic brain injury, due to the life changes, setbacks, and differences we deal with on a daily basis. Most people do not understand what we go through each day, but I do not blame any of them. Everyone—I mean everyone—has "stuff" to deal with. Life gives all of us challenges, but we do not get to choose which ones we receive and attempt to overcome. We have been through so much, but it definitely is not over yet."

Extending Compassion

It's certainly true that everyone has their own "stuff" they are dealing with. Everyone's individual battle is the one that matters most to them—and rightfully so. *There is more than enough compassion to go around,* so let's all try to be a bit more compassionate to one another, even if we don't fully understand that person's invisible injury, or whatever it is they are going through at the time. Friendships may ebb and flow, but a simple "thinking of you" text, email, call, or card can go a long way in boosting someone's morale and helping in her recovery.

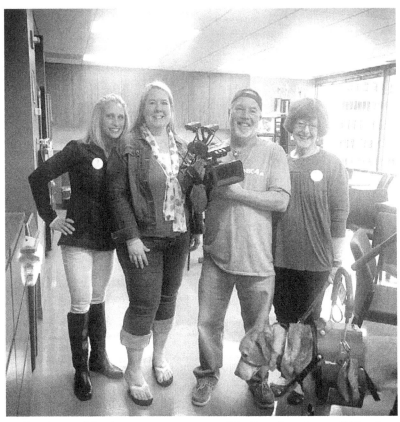

Posing with the cameraman with Stephanie and Toni after an interview with "NBC Washington."

Chapter Four

Quit Using Your Brain Injury
As An Excuse

August 2016

66*Quit using your brain injury as an excuse!"*
     I was caught completely off guard by this statement
a few weeks ago, said by someone I have known many
years. She had followed my TBI story, and I thought she
had an understanding of what I was going through.
Apparently, I was wrong.

We had been talking, and I had to ask her to repeat what
she said a bit earlier. When I did, she looked at me and
said, "You know, Amy. You really need to stop using your
brain injury as an excuse. You're starting to use it as a
crutch."

Wait, WHAT?!

I wanted to scream, "ARE YOU KIDDING?? This is a
joke, right?"

But I didn't. I kept my composure and explained to her
how it's not an excuse or a crutch—*it's my "new normal,"*
and that she doesn't understand the pain it causes me to
know that this is how life is now. I further explained the
part of my brain that was damaged now causes me to have

difficulty remembering things in the short-term, and I often confuse words and forget meanings.

Why on earth would I ask her to repeat something if I didn't really need her to? She explained that she thought I wasn't focused enough—and I should "try harder" to remember things.

I about fell off my chair.

I actually have to try twice as hard to follow a conversation as I did before my brain injury.

One of my biggest struggles two-and-a-half years after my TBI is my short-term memory. I have to pay extra attention, and sometimes get confused by words I "should" know the meaning of but have forgotten, which is part of the *aphasia*.

I realize that before my injury I was a focused, independent, strong-willed woman. I was full of con-fidence, and my peers looked to me for advice. I understand it's hard for those peers to understand exactly what I am going through—but to actually tell me I'm using my brain injury as an excuse, and I "just" need to try harder and focus more, well, that is simply plain ignorance.

It is frustrating to vividly remember the woman I once was, the woman who could remember a 30-item shopping list, and multitask with ease. Those days are long gone, for now. I am hopeful my memory will continue to improve, and my cognitive function comes back to full capacity. But for now, *I am who I am.*

*Terry from Edmonton, Alberta, Canada wrote:
"When someone implies I am faking, I feel alone,
wrongly accused, and frustrated with that
person's lack of knowledge and understanding."*

I am on a mission to help educate those who are not
familiar with the long-term effects of brain injury.

We hear celebrities like comedian Tracy Morgan
express that he is 100 percent back to normal one year
after a horrific car accident, when in reality, these types of
recoveries are extremely rare. Most recoveries take
years—and are almost never 100 percent complete.
Perhaps he is putting on a positive front, and I wonder
whether Morgan is actually 100 percent recovered. Those
closest to him are likely to notice he still has speech and
memory issues, in addition to neuro-fatigue.

*Lauren from Pennsylvania puts it so eloquently:
"I have to embrace my 'new normal' to the best of
my ability or else I will be lying to myself and get
nowhere. With the support of the people in my life,
mindfulness, spiritual awareness and a never-
give-up attitude, I am able to enlighten others with
awareness of the huge shift that is now my life. I
would be lying to say it's as easy as black and
white, because it is not. I must remember to
ground myself and to prove only to myself that I
am going to be okay."*

I have (almost) completely accepted this "new me" who has memory and word issues, and cognitive impairments. I regularly hear from other survivors about how they feel so isolated and alone because their friends and family don't understand what they're going through.

I understand I am in this for the long haul. I wish those around me would show more compassion and make an attempt at understanding.

It is frustrating that we have to stuff our anger inside when someone says something like, "Quit using your brain injury as an excuse." Yet, I also know lashing out at them with anger doesn't solve anything. So the next time someone says something like this to me, *I am going to simply respond with: "I am so sorry you feel that way."*

To those who do not completely understand, and thus think we're making excuses, please know that recovery can take *years*—and may never be full and complete.

Next time you're tempted to imply we're making excuses, understand that most survivors will be left with a combination of these symptoms:

- Short-term memory loss
- Trouble focusing our attention
- Neuro-fatigue (running out of energy)
- Dizziness and balance issues
- Cognitive deficits (processing things slower than before)
- Aphasia (trouble recalling or understanding words)

- Not being able to handle overstimulation (lots of people, light, and noise)
- Anxiety about the simplest things
- Depression
- Chronic pain

In short, we are *not* making excuses, we are simply doing the best we can with what we have been given. All of us want to get back to work, back to a meaningful life, back to the way we were before our injury. It's a long, lonely road, which is not made easier by other people's ignorance. *Remember, compassion makes the world go around.*

I have a brain injury, *what's your excuse?*

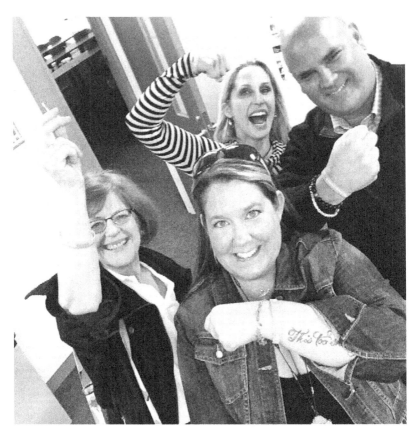

Toni, Stephanie, Paul, and I showing off our TBI
Awareness wristbands at Argosy University in
Washington, D.C.

Chapter Five

Four Lessons I Learned From NASCAR About Concussions

August 2016

I have been following Dale Earnhardt, Jr.'s recovery since he sustained a concussion in a June 12 crash at Michigan International Speedway. In July, Earnhardt was diag-nosed with concussion-like symptoms and announced he would miss the second half of the year as a result.

Dale Jr. regularly updated his fans about his recovery via Twitter, Instagram, and Facebook Live, and *I admire his open and honest account* of his symptoms and recovery regimens.

In one video, he takes you on his journey to the grocery store where he admits he is suffering from anxiety and overstimulation, which are some of the most *invisible and misunderstood* symptoms of concussion.

These videos are so relatable to anyone who has suffered a concussion, and I applaud Dale Jr. for taking the initiative to simultaneously help others who are going through similar experiences, while educating the general public about the invisible "stuff" that lurks under the surface, unseen by the outsider.

Additionally, NASCAR has been outstanding in their handling of Dale Jr.'s situation. Nothing but positivity and support has come from his team and the NASCAR association.

Here are four racing metaphor lessons I have learned from NASCAR:

1. **Take Yourself Out of the Race**
   Don't get back into the car again until you're cleared to race (literally and figuratively). It's not worth the risk, because you're putting your own life in danger, as well as those around you.
2. **Watch for the "Caution Flag"**
   Listen to your doctor, understand your symptoms, and be diligent about your recovery therapies. Remember symptoms can vary from person to person, and accident to accident. No two concussions or recoveries are the same.
3. **Celebrate the Victories**
   Celebrate the small victories in your recovery. Like Dale Jr.'s grocery store outing, it's the little things that make us aware of the symptoms, and keep us moving forward in our recoveries. Sure, there will be setbacks and bad days, so always cherish the good days.
4. **Know Your Position**
   With every sport and activity we participate in, there is always a chance for concussion. Understanding the risks and being aware of the

symptoms is key in getting proper treatment—and getting it as quickly as possible.

Earnhardt has stated he eventually wants to get back on the racetrack, but for *right now his focus is on healing and getting better.* He is taking his recovery seriously and putting racing on the back burner until he is cleared to race again.

NOTE: On December 8, 2016, Earnhardt was medically cleared to return to competition in 2017, but he then announced he would retire at the end of the 2017 season—which he did.

What Earnhardt's public statements say to the world is "this happened to me," and "this is how it affected me." His words help enlighten the public to the possible symptoms anyone with a concussion may have, and empower the more than 2.8 million Americans who will suffer a brain injury each year.

Knowledge is power, and brings about understanding, patience, and empathy in others.

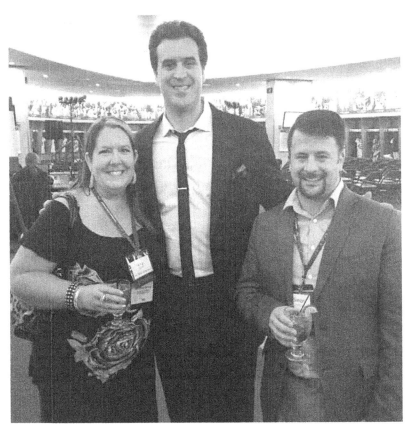

Simon and I meeting NFL Super Bowl Champ, Ben Utecht, at
the "Standing Strong" fundraiser for the American
Brain Foundation.

Chapter Six

Ben Utecht, NFL Champ, Writes Book About Concussions And Memory Loss

August 2016

> *"It took losing my mind to care about my mind."*
> – Ben Utecht

B en Utecht is best known for his role as Super Bowl champion tight end for the Indianapolis Colts, playing alongside quarterback Peyton Manning. In addition to his football career, he is also a gifted musician, loving hus-band, and a dedicated father to four beautiful girls.

You can now add "author" to his list of talents, as Utecht released his first book, *Counting the Days While My Mind Slips Away: A Love Letter to My Fam*ily. In this book he chronicles his remarkable journey, and how he is losing his memories as the result of multiple concussions sustained during his days playing football in college and the NFL.

In our interview, Ben told me at its core, his book is a memoir, an opportunity for him to chronicle his football story, as well as the story of meeting his wife and births of his daughters—so he has a way to tell his daughters about it, in case one day he no longer remembers any of it.

His first football concussion occurred during college while playing for the University of Minnesota. In the book, he states he felt groggy and disoriented as the coaches helped him to his feet. One of the trainers said, "You have a concussion, that's all. It sure looked like it could have been something bad."

Utecht goes on to explain, "Unless someone got knocked out cold, like I did, we never even thought of these injuries as concussions. We all just referred to them as getting our bell rung, or getting lit up." Ben was cleared to return to play the following week.

While playing four years of college and five years of NFL football, Ben would have a total of five documented concussions.

After his fourth concussion, he had amnesia for a short period, and Ben noticed his memory was getting fuzzy and his cognitive skills were a bit slow—none of which he mentioned to anyone. In his previous incidents, he had always returned to play by the next week, but this one was harder for him to shake. He kept failing his ImPACT tests, but would eventually return to play a few weeks later.

NOTE: Trusted by sports teams, schools, corporations, hospitals, and clinics, ImPACT is the most widely used computerized neurocognitive test used to help evaluate and manage concussions.

In his book Ben writes:

> I finally passed the ImPACT test in time to practice for the Jaguars' game. In my mind, and in the eyes of the team medical staff, passing the test meant I was over the concussion, that I was back to my old self. I wasn't. When asked when I finally felt normal again, I don't think I ever I did. I have never been the same since the first quarter of the fourth game of my fourth NFL season. Eight years later and counting, I now realize the person I was before is never coming back.

I have to confess while reading Ben's book, many instances made me cringe. Having suffered a severe concussion myself after falling on a patch of ice, I can't even begin to fathom getting back out on the field and playing a week later. Reading about his headaches, dizziness, slowed cognitive thinking, and memory loss, it all profoundly resonated with me.

In August 2009, he suffered a career-ending concussion during pre-season practice with the Cincinnati Bengals. When the team called to tell his wife, Karyn, he had suffered another concussion, she actually breathed a sigh of relief that it wasn't more serious. She still had what was then the common mindset that *a concussion was no big deal.*

While Ben was on the injured reserve, he continually tried to improve his condition, without much success.

Doctors wouldn't clear him to return to play this time, and his headaches and memory were becoming worse. He would eventually receive the phone call every player dreads—he had been cut from the team. His career was essentially over at the age of 28.

Ben told me writing this book was therapeutic, and a very emotional process. He had a number of challenges along the way, and his family had to help him with many of the details because so many of his memories were completely gone.

> *I am not a bitter man, I love football. I want to see it done the right way, at all levels. I want to tell a story that makes people consider, for the first time maybe, how critical their mind is to their identity. If that shifts as a culture, that will have a great impact on the brain health of athletes.* – Ben Utecht

His message to parents is simple:
- Educate yourself fully, understand what a concussion injury and its symptoms are, and what to do if it happens to your child.
- If you want your children to play sports, build a relationship with a neurologist and get a baseline assessment of your child.
- Understand that between the ages of 2 and 12 is when your child's brain is going through the most growth and developmental changes.

- Don't enter your child into sports until after age 12.

Ben also understands the importance of athletics, and how it affects many youth. Being a part of a team is important for gaining leadership skills and responsibility. Ben admits having four daughters is a bit of relief, knowing they will likely never want to play football. He hopes they follow in their mother's footsteps and take up golf.

He hopes sharing his story will help spread a message on the importance of our memory and brain health. Speaking and giving leadership programs has become Ben's passion, "Speaking is about influencing just one." It's not about how many people you're in front of, it's the impact your words can have, even if it's just one person—because that one person could turn your message into something for millions. You never know when you're going to be the miracle for somebody."

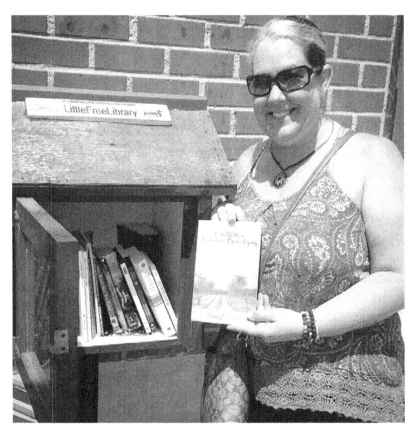

Leaving my book at a "Little Free Library" in Brentwood Village, Los Angeles, California.

Chapter Seven

Let's Talk About Sex...After Brain Injury

October 2016

> *"Sexual energy is the primal and creative energy of the universe."*
>
> — Deepak Chopra

Five reasons why my sex drive changed after a traumatic brain injury

As someone who had a fairly healthy sex drive before falling on the ice and suffering a traumatic brain injury (TBI), I was confused as to what was going on with my libido.

It's a story I hear far too often among TBI survivors: *they want* to be intimate with their partner, yet don't have the bandwidth to even consider it. The partner feels neglected and/or frustrated, and the survivor feels helpless and misunderstood. This cycle can continue for years, and I felt it was time to speak out on a topic that affects over 2.8 million Americans each year, yet is rarely talked about: Sex After Brain Injury.

For the past few years I have had a "friends-with-benefits" situation with Tim (not his real name.) We enjoy each other's company, and have a great sexual chemistry together. He lives about an hour west of the Twin Cities, so I see him only every few months, which works out perfectly for both of us.

I saw Tim several times in the first few months after my fall and it was, well, *interesting*. In addition to a TBI, I had also sustained whiplash, torn muscles, and a dislocated sternum. *Finding a position for me to get comfortable in was challenging, to say the least.* Tim was patient with me, and very gentle and kind. He understood my situation and wanted to do whatever he could to make it easier for me.

It was almost comical, the amount of work it took— propping me up on pillows so I wouldn't be dizzy, repositioning me every few minutes so I wouldn't be in pain, and let's not forget I couldn't "jiggle" my head around or it would cause an instant headache.

After Tim's first two visits, I simply wasn't even interested in sex anymore. Not because it took too much work, but because *I didn't have the energy.* I didn't even have the desire to "make out," and even giving him a hug took everything I had. When Tim would stop by for a visit, I would basically sit on the couch in a zombie-like state while we talked about the weather. It was awkward, but he never made me feel bad, although I am sure he was disappointed.

His visits became less frequent, but we still talked often on the phone. Fortunately, we had a good friendship, and the "benefits" were only part of the deal.

About two years after my fall, I was expecting a visit from Tim and was actually looking forward to it. I felt I was ready to give an afternoon romp another try. Alas, I had a killer headache when he showed up. He could tell just by looking at me, and hearing the difficulty I had speaking— that a romp *was not* going to happen.

I was so frustrated because I had actually psyched myself up enough to *want* to have sex again. It was the first time in almost two years I had felt the need inside of me. I knew how good we were together in the bedroom, and wanted to experience that feeling of intimacy with him again.

He recently came to town again, and this time I was determined to make it happen. Finally, after two and a half years, Amy was ready for "sexy time" again. I still struggled with a bit of dizziness, but I powered through it, and didn't let it distract me. I reassured Tim I was ready to try this or that, and we had a fun afternoon together.

I had missed the feeling of intimacy, almost as much as I missed my memory and spunky personality.

While most of my physical injuries have healed, every inch of my body hurt the following day. It took me a few days to recover physically and restore my energy levels, but it was completely worth it...*Amy got her groove back!* Tim commented on the fact he could tell my personality was returning to "normal," and was happy to see me feeling more energetic and lively.

While I am fortunate my "friend with benefits" was compassionate and understanding, I completely understand how relationships are turned upside down by TBI. Not only is the person and his or her partner dealing with an invisible injury, the partner is also getting frustrated with what is *and isn't* happening in the bedroom. While the person may be physically back to normal, she or he is still dealing with a lot of the invisible symptoms of TBI.

From my experience, I've learned five main areas of my TBI were holding my body back from having a sex drive:

1. **Neuro-Fatigue.** Our energy levels are severely limited after a brain injury. Every single thing we do throughout the day requires energy. Whether it's brushing our teeth, reading emails, going for a walk, or washing the dishes, we are taking energy from our reserves. We are easily tired, and although I sleep ten hours at night, I still require a two-hour nap during the afternoon. The thought of trying to add sex into my daily routine was daunting, and I'm sure if I had a spouse or partner, he would have been frustrated. However, it is important for the partner to understand it's not him (or her), and it has absolutely *nothing* to do with him—and it could take a long time to get our energy levels and stamina back. It took me two and a half years to be ready to participate in a single afternoon of lovemaking.

2. **Dizziness and Balance Issues.** Many brain injury survivors suffer from being dizzy and having balance disorders. In the early days after my TBI, I couldn't lie flat on my back, nor could I bend over without practically passing out. While one can try a lot of positions in the bedroom, almost all of them caused some degree of dizziness. Circle back to my first point about neuro-fatigue, when combined with the already-tired brain with some dizziness, it's a recipe for disaster.

3. **Chronic Pain.** Not all brain injury survivors will have other physical injuries, but I did. Even two and a half years later, I still deal with a lot of chronic pain. In the bedroom it hurt my chest, neck, and shoulders to be on the top, bottom, or anywhere in between. Again, think of neuro-fatigue, coupled with chronic pain...are you starting to get the picture?

4. **Apathy.** Having a total lack of interest in *anything*—not just sex—is one of the most common side effects of a brain injury. I remember my personality being "flat" for the first two years, and wondering if I would ever laugh again, or want to do any of my hobbies again. I can't say it too often: *every single thing we do takes energy.* I think our brains instinctively try to preserve as much energy as possible, and having an interest in something is *a low priority.* I remember not wanting to do pretty

much anything. Laundry and cooking were horrific tasks, as was driving to my favorite store.

5. **Overstimulation.** Let's be real: sex involves *a lot of stimulation*. Even a healthy, active person without a brain injury can readily admit that sex engages pretty much every one of our senses to an extreme. Our brains are already running on conserved energy. I remember worrying I was going to stroke-out the first time I had sex after my TBI. My heart was racing out of control, my head was pounding, I was dizzy, my entire body hurt, and all the while I was trying to make sure my partner wasn't aware of the hell going on inside my head.

    Even going out to eat at a loud and people-filled restaurant is a major undertaking with all the background noise and lights, and people talking. Is there any wonder having sex is just too much for our brains?

I hope having read this far, you are gaining a better understanding into the struggle of living with a brain injury.

I also hope...

- If you are the survivor, you give yourself grace, and know you're not alone in the journey.
- If you're the partner, you can have a better understanding of what the other person is going through. While I can't even imagine how

frustrating this has to be for you, it's ten times more frustrating for the survivor.

While I know I got my sexual groove back, it's going to be different for every single person. It's important for both of you to be patient and understanding, and for the partner to be compassionate and empathetic. And most importantly for both of you...enjoy just being there with your loved one.

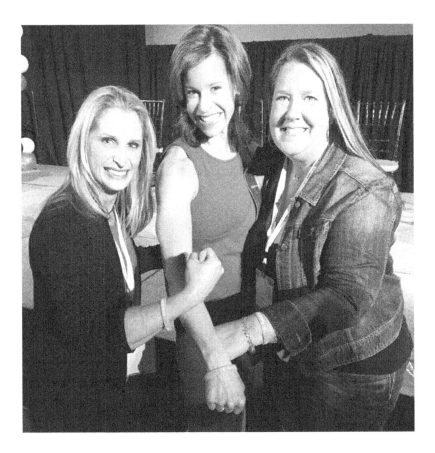

Stephanie and I meeting with Jenna Wolfe from "The Jenna Wolfe Show," sporting our TBI Awareness bracelets in Washington, D.C.

Chapter Eight

Five Symptoms of PTSD After Brain Injury

December 2016

As I near the three-year anniversary of my traumatic brain injury (TBI), I am once again reminded of how fragile I still am.

My TBI was the result of a slip and fall on an icy driveway in February 2014. I had zero warning as my feet slipped out from under me, and my skull took the full impact of my fall. *I can still* hear the god-awful sound of my skull hitting the pavement.

About nine months after my fall, I suffered an extreme panic attack. I had never suffered from any form of anxiety before my accident, other than the occasional butterflies before a big presentation, etc. I honestly thought I was having a heart attack because my heart was racing *so* fast— and I couldn't get it under control with breathing techniques.

Later my chiropractic neurologist referred me to a therapist who specializes in PTSD (post-traumatic stress disorder) and chronic pain. He quickly pieced together that my panic attack stemmed from the fact we had just received our first snow and ice of the new winter season, and my body/brain was reacting to the emotional trauma now stored inside me from my fall on the ice.

What a relief to know there was a "reason" I was experiencing such extreme anxiety and distress, and thus it became easier to get it under control when I knew what was causing it.

I would eventually work with a physical therapist who specializes in cranial sacral therapy. During one of our sessions, he explained how our bodies store the emotional trauma of whatever we have been through—even if our minds don't remember the event. Like for me, I couldn't actually remember the fall and hitting my head, only the sound it made.

The therapist explained how PTSD is common with any form of assault, and essentially, I had been assaulted *by the pavement.* When he worded it like that, it was *like a light bulb went on.* That was exactly how I felt, but hadn't been able to pinpoint it.

Recently I found a functional neurologist who has helped me tremendously with many of my symptoms, including my PTSD and anxiety. One of the techniques he used was to put me on a tilt table, and move me into almost the exact position, duplicating how I landed when my feet first went out from under me. I started crying the first time he positioned me there. He would then put me into this position again, and draw letters on the bottom of my feet and ask me to name the letter, while at the same time using an electric stimulator on my ankle. It was amazing how the anxiety melted away.

I have been fortunate to find professionals who truly understand PTSD, anxiety, and brain injury. Many survivors struggle to find anyone who will actually listen, and who do not rule them out *as faking or malingering*.

> According to Wikipedia: PTSD was originally classified as a mental disorder, but has recently been reclassified as a "trauma- and stressor-related disorder." The characteristic symptoms were not present before exposure to the traumatic event, and while it is common to have symptoms after any traumatic event, these must persist to a certain degree for longer than one month after the trauma to be classified as PTSD. Causes of the symptoms of PTSD are the experiencing or witnessing of a stressor event involving death, serious injury, or such threat to the self or others in a situation in which the individual felt intense fear, horror, or powerlessness.

Sad but true, friends and family don't understand brain injury, and if you combine that with PTSD and anxiety, it's a recipe for extreme stress. I get it—if you have never experienced anxiety or trauma to your body, it *is* hard to understand. But...it is not hard to offer compassion and a shoulder to cry on for support. The last thing we need is someone judging us for something that is very real and terrifying. We are doing the best we can to survive day-to-day tasks, and could really use all the support we can get.

While I am not a therapist, I have found five common symptoms that I—and my fellow TBI survivors—have experienced.

1. **Anxiety at the scene of the initial accident.** I am almost three years out from my accident, and I still have a hard time walking down that same driveway, even on a dry, sunny summer day. Once snow and ice cover it, I actually cry when I have to walk down it, and I become paralyzed with fear.

2. **Fear of hurting oneself again.** I go through periods of time where I have an irrational fear of accidentally hurting myself again (not only from a fall in the driveway). These thoughts usually creep in as our temperatures start to drop, and the threat of snow and ice comes into the forecast. I *worry* about hitting my head on the open cupboard door, or of being in a car accident, or any other scenario my brain conjures up.

3. **Flashbacks or nightmares.** In the beginning I regularly had flashbacks of my fall. They have subsided, but still surface when we start to get ice and snow. I notice I also have more nightmares during this time of year, and they mostly involve getting hurt. I occasionally startle myself awake when I hear my skull impacting with the pavement.

4. **Difficulty talking about the traumatic event.**
   Early on I had an extremely hard time opening up
   about my accident, but have since found it quite
   therapeutic to write and speak about it—and I know
   I am helping others through my work. Many survivors find those who have not experienced a brain
   injury, or any form of anxiety, simply can't
   understand what we are dealing with, and will often
   dismiss our feelings, which certainly causes even
   more anxiety.

5. **Self-isolation.** Because many survivors feel misunderstood, we choose not to attend social gather-
   ings. I also find I don't want to leave the comfort of
   my home when there is ice and snow covering the
   sidewalks and roads. It is as if we go into self-
   protection mode...and hibernate.

I am enveloped in fear and anxiety when I walk on snow
and ice, and whether it's an intersection where you had
your car accident, or the hospital where you had brain
surgery, the scene of your accident can be a constant
trigger for anxiety.

I am beyond lucky to have found medical professionals
who have helped me to understand my PTSD and to keep
it in check. I strongly urge you to seek a therapist who
specializes in PTSD and/or brain injury. Seeing a therapist
does not make you "weak" or mean that you have "mental
problems."

Not all therapists are created equal, and if at first you don't find one you like, keep searching until you find the right fit. I was lucky, and found a great one right away.

Nothing is more reassuring and validating than to have someone tell you that you are indeed "normal" for experiencing the anxiety, fear, and thoughts you have after a traumatic brain injury. It is part of the healing process.

While I am always caught off guard by the fact that my PTSD still exists, each winter when the weather changes to arctic, I am reminded how fragile we truly are. We are human, and we are survivors!

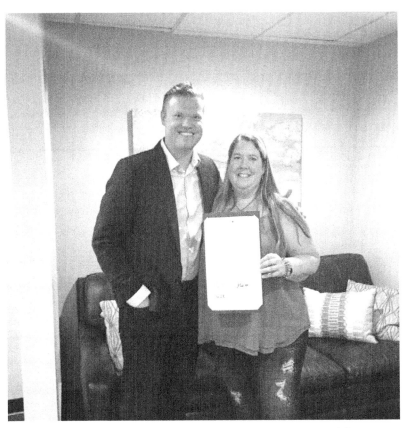

Celebrating Concussion Awareness Day with
Dr. Jeremy Schmoe.

Chapter Nine

How Functional Neurology Helped Improve My Quality of Life After Brain Injury

January 2017

As we begin the new year, I am reflecting on all for which I have to be grateful. Toward the top of that list is finally finding Dr. Jeremy Schmoe, DC, DACNB, a functional neurologist who has been instrumental in helping me rehab my brain injury.

Going Back...

Immediately after my fall, I used a chiropractic neurologist who helped me with my whiplash, torn muscles, and dislocated sternum. He diagnosed me as having a severe concussion, and told me I should start feeling better in about four to six weeks.

I kept complaining that I felt my eyes weren't quite right, and I was experiencing a lot of short-term memory problems and aphasia, as well as major dizziness and balance issues. He eventually sent me to a neurologist who didn't seem to believe my issues were a problem (even though I couldn't touch my nose with my pointer finger). When I later read her reports, I had to laugh. She had stated I was dressed nicely and was well groomed, where in fact I hadn't showered in days and was wearing the same yoga pants and sweatshirt I had been wearing for about three days. Had she asked, I would have outright admitted this to her.

She eventually sent me for a *neuropsychological exam* to measure my deficits. After a grueling four-hour test designed to make me face my weaknesses, I scheduled a meeting with the neuropsychologist the following week. She very kindly explained to me the nature of the test, how it measures deficits, and how it is essentially "fake proof." She then implied I must have been faking because I scored too poorly in memory, and my scores were lower than a patient with dementia. After spending about 70 minutes with me, she assessed I should be put on Ritalin, anti-depressants, and sleep medication.

I refused all three because I knew they wouldn't actually "heal" me, and would be only a temporary crutch.

I had been begging every neuro doctor I saw for help. I didn't know what type of therapy I needed, but I knew I needed something—cognitive, occupational, vision, anything that would help me get back to the person I used to be. The dizziness was sucking all the life out of me, and the short-term memory problems were causing quite a challenge to function in every-day settings.

I was incredibly frustrated as I went back to my neurologist about a year later. After a brief assessment, she told me that because it was over a year since my injury, none of the therapies would likely help me. WHAT?? Then why on earth didn't she send me earlier? I was confused, frust-rated, and felt hopeless.

As a last resort, the neurologist did eventually send me to a cranial sacral therapist who was the first person to help me find any sort of relief. His gentle treatment helped realign the skull plates that had been causing pressure inside my head. After several treatments, I felt a lot of relief from the "brain fog" that had been a 24/7 nuisance.

After two and a half years of struggling through life with a brain injury, Dr. Jeremy Schmoe of Minnesota Functional Neurology in Minneapolis reached out to me. He had read several of my *HuffPost* articles, and noticed we both lived in the metro area. His message said he knew he could help me, and wanted me to come in for an exam.

To be honest, I brushed him off for a while. Every doctor I had seen up to this point had discouraged me, and my neurologist told me there was basically no hope for further recovery—even though I had learned that recovery can happen at any point after your injury.

To Dr. Schmoe's credit, he was persistent, and I eventually agreed to go in for a consultation. I figured it was worth a shot—and I had nothing to lose.

My initial exam took almost two hours and consisted of checking my:

- Balance
- Gait
- Heart rate and blood pressure
- Visual eye tracking (VNG)
- Quick eye movements (saccades)
- Optokinetic reflexes (OPK)
- Vestibular Ocular Reflexes (VOR)
- Chiropractic structural examination

My testing showed the following results:

- My autonomic nervous system was too sympathetic (startle response).
- My resting heart rate was too high.
- My gaze-holding ability was questionable.
- All planes of my smooth pursuit eye movements were impaired.
- I was unsteady standing on flat surfaces, and would fall backward when I closed my eyes.
- Spatial awareness and depth perception were impaired.
- My walking gait was impaired.
- I had diminished sensation on the left side of my face and body.
- My visual and auditory reaction times were off.

Dr. Schmoe had validated *every single thing I had been feeling.*

He said we needed to work on all of the systems *together* in order to get them working properly again. He told me the majority of my issues were coming from my eyes, and we needed to retrain my eyes how to work properly. It was so comforting to know I wasn't crazy at all—it was just that those other doctors had been ignoring all of my issues because they weren't trained in what to look for related to traumatic brain injuries and concussions. I have learned first-hand this is widely misunderstood by medical professionals.

> *Functional neurology is a way of thinking and assessing the nervous system* by looking at what's working well, what isn't working, and what might be working too much. It's about developing strategies to build better plasticity in how your nervous system is working.

Dr. Schmoe believes functional neurology should be a basic requirement in all medical and healthcare fields, but unfortunately it is not.

Dr. Schmoe gained his knowledge by attending the Carrick Institute for those who have already graduated from the chiropractic program. The Carrick Institute program is an additional three years of training beyond chiropractic school. It is designed to give a deeper education and understanding of how the nervous system works, and how to treat problems that arise as the result of a brain injury or disease. They offer courses to providers of all disciplines, including medical doctors, physical therapists, naturopaths, etc.

Dr. Schmoe gave me treatment plans for each of my systems that weren't working, which included:

- Gaze-stability exercises and vestibular rehab
- Tilt table with electric stimulation to calm my startle reflex
- Sensory stimulation on the left side of my body
- Finger-to-nose cerebellum training on the left side
- ARP wave simulation on my neck (whiplash)
- Doctor-applied FNOR techniques on my shoulder and scapula
- FNOR physical rehabilitation exercises to strengthen neck, core, and lower extremities
- Prologel to lessen inflammation in my neck from my whiplash that hadn't healed
- D2 exercises to increase my hand-eye reaction times
- Interactive metronome exercises to increase my auditory reaction times
- Blood chemistry workup to check for anemia, infections, inflammation, autoimmune disorders, thyroid and blood sugar levels
- Dietary and nutrition supplements

Within only two weeks of working on gaze-stabilization and eye-tracking exercises, I was no longer feeling dizzy and off-balance. Dealing with dizziness 24/7 was a major energy suck, and I was starting to notice I now had more energy to get things done during the day than I had had since my accident.

I was starting to gain back feeling in the left side of my body, and my startle response was settling down. As a result of all of this, my anxiety levels were diminishing. It's amazing how your body responds when you are no longer constantly living in a high-pain threshold. I was finally able to go several weeks without a headache, which was great since I had been having headaches on an all-too-regular basis.

Now this isn't to say I am "fixed"…I still have a long way to go. But I am finally feeling better than I have since February 2014. If Dr. Schmoe had found me a year earlier, who knows where I would be in my recovery right now.

It astounds me how one doctor could improve so many of my symptoms with "simple" techniques, yet a plethora of trained neurological doctors *didn't do anything for me.* This is why I am so passionate about the advocacy work I do. Millions of brain injury survivors have not had proper treatment, and are basically disregarded by the medical community—and written off by the psychologists as having "mental" issues rather than "physical" issues.

Some professionals have gone so far as to say now universally "everyone has a brain injury," as a result of the media talking about concussions and sports. The reality is that we are only beginning to understand the severity of concussions, and people who were injured decades ago are just beginning to understand why they've felt and acted the way they have for so many years—as their brain injury went undiagnosed.

With proper treatment, the brain and neurological system has an amazing way of rewiring itself. The key is early detection and diagnosis, in combination with a trained doctor who understands how to best treat you, and not brush you off or disregard your concerns.

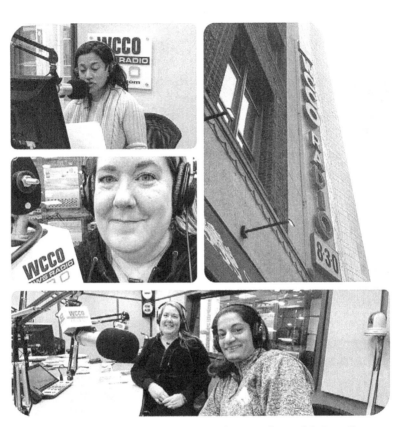

Hanging out with Dr. Uzma Samadani and Roshini Rajkumar at the WCCO radio station in Minneapolis during a recent interview.

Chapter Ten

Eye Movements May Be Key In Detecting Brain Injury, Concussion

August 2017

D r. Uzma Samadani, M.D., Ph.D., is paving the way for new eye-tracking diagnostic measures after a brain injury.

I had the pleasure of hearing Dr. Uzma Samadani speak at a Minnesota Brain Injury Alliance conference for professionals, and was mesmerized by what she had to share regarding eye-tracking and the correlation to brain injury. I couldn't soak up enough of what she had to share that day, so I was ecstatic to have the opportunity to interview her for an article, and you might say I was even a little star-struck.

You see, eye-tracking was my biggest complaint, and no one bothered to acknowledge it.

Immediately after my fall that resulted in my traumatic brain injury (TBI), I knew my eyes weren't quite right. In the beginning I wasn't even able to read the words on my computer screen, like when I was trying to find the local ER. Time passed, and I kept telling every doctor I saw that *something wasn't quite right* with my eyes.

Eventually I was sent to a neuro-ophthalmologist who did extensive testing, only to tell me my eyes were "fine." I continued struggling with my vision and went to my eye doctor, who has known me for over ten years. She tried everything to help me, and concluded I was seeing double, and my left eye was trying extra hard to keep me from seeing double, therefore causing strain on my eye.

It was the best answer I had been given thus far, yet I still didn't feel it was good enough.

I was convinced my eyes were causing my dizziness and balance issues, and everyone blew me off by saying it was just positional vertigo. When I would go to sleep at night, I could feel my eyes start to move around on their own. However, I was dismissed over and over, indicating I was imagining it, and I was suffering from positional vertigo.

This is *not* what was affecting me.

At the two-and-a-half-year mark Dr. Jeremy Schmoe, from Minnesota Functional Neurology DC in Minneapolis, reached out to me after reading one of my *HuffPost* blogs. He told me he was confident he would be able to help me with my dizziness and balance issues.

I was skeptical at first because everyone else blew me off—and had never really listened to me.

At my initial consultation, Dr. Schmoe spent two hours with me performing all sorts of tests. One of the very first tests he did was to run a red-and-white striped pattern past me, telling me to focus on only the white squares. The second he moved it, I had a dizzy spell and had to look away.

His response? "It's your eyes. They're not moving together properly."

I wanted to cry, but this time it was happy tears instead of frustrated tears. Finally, someone seemed to understand that my eyes indeed were causing me problems.

Dr. Schmoe explained, "You can sometimes evaluate eye movements, and the eye muscle and vision can look fine, but when the brain has to deal with a complex sensory environment, and the mechanisms to compensate have been injured, this can be a terrifying situation. In your case, there was involvement of all three systems (cervical, visual, and vestibular) which lead to sensory confusion or mismatch in the brain, causing horrific symptoms and changes in your autonomic system and emotionality."

Now when I was talking to Dr. Samadani, she considers it complete serendipity that she began the study of eye-tracking. She had finished her residency and was conducting clinical trials for brain injury when a colleague suggested using eye-tracking as an outcome measure.

They began working on their technology, now known as EyeBOX™, in the summer of 2011, and applied for their first patent in 2012, which was issued in spring 2017. The study of elevated intracranial pressure (ICP) and reversible eye-tracking began in 2014, and was funded by a NASA-affiliate organization interested in helping astronauts achieve prolonged space travel. Astronauts develop visual and cognitive problems while in space deployment, which mimics elevated intracranial pressure on earth, and NASA wanted to find a way to detect this.

Dr. Samadani explained a concussion can disrupt eye movements in at least two ways: 1) through elevating intracranial pressure, and 2) by physiological disruption of neurologic pathways—not bad enough that pressure goes up, but it causes irritation.

In the study, a patient watches a music video on a computer screen that contains a square moving around the screen. As a patient follows the square, the device measures eye coordination. The device is attached to the computer so a patient doesn't have to wear it on his or her head.

When Dr. Samadani's team developed their device, they wanted to make sure a patient who wasn't able to follow instructions would still be capable of using it. "Essentially, we are testing brain stem function, which is done involuntarily, meaning you don't have to think about it," stated Samadani.

Historically, measuring the nerves that move the eye has been done by having a patient look in a direction, like up, down, left, right; however, that assumes a certain amount of function.

Eventually Dr. Samadani discovered the equipment could ultimately detect differences in the left and right eye movements. The test does not need a baseline since 98.78 percent of people's eyes move together.

The recent study looking at elevated intracranial pressure (ICP) included 23 patients who required intracranial pressure monitoring for clinical reasons, including bleeding in the brain, while others were being monitored for pressure due to tumor or stroke. The study showed nerve function in the brain decreased when pressure was elevated, and returned to normal when it came back down. The effect of elevated ICP on nerve function was detectable within minutes of ICP elevation.

Reviews by optometrists have shown as many as 90 percent of people who seek attention for their concussion/brain injury have eye-tracking problems.

Dr. Samadani's team hopes this device will help patients receive the proper care right away, saying, "We want someone who has suffered a traumatic brain injury to be diagnosed as quickly as possible so they can be treated appropriately."

She concluded by saying, "The majority of people who hit their heads don't have a brain injury; however, we want to help identify those who need treatment."

About Dr. Samadani: Dr. Uzma Samadani founded Oculogica in 2013, and her laboratory has developed the eye-tracking methodology and published six papers on its utility. She is currently the Rockswold Kaplan Endowed Chair for Traumatic Brain Injury at Hennepin County Medical Center and Associate Professor of Neurosurgery at the University of Minnesota. She serves on the American Association of Neurological Surgeons/Congress of Neurological Surgeons Executive Committee for

Trauma and Critical Care and is Scientific Program Chair of the AANS/CNS National Neurotrauma Society Joint Satellite Meeting.

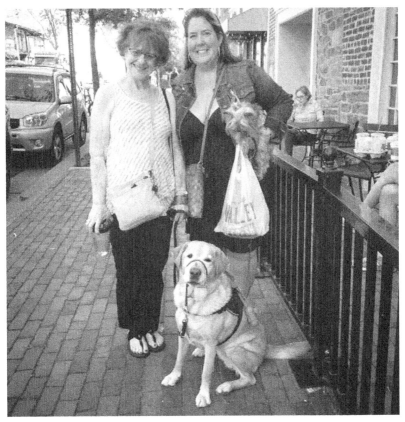

Pixxie and I hanging out with Toni and Bud in Virginia.

Chapter Eleven

A Struggle Back to Financial Freedom
After a Brain Injury

March 2017

While in a coma, Harvey lost his civil rights *and* all control over his own money, due to a court-ordered conservator-ship. A durable power of attorney could have prevented this nightmare situation.

On a beautiful June day in 2009, Harvey was riding his motorcycle up the Pacific Coast Highway (PCH) in Malibu as he had many times before. He enjoyed the scenery and the feel of the open road. However, he has almost zero memory of this particular day.

As he neared the Malibu Pier, a woman driving a sedan ahead of him suddenly made an illegal U-turn, turning directly into his motorcycle. The highway was shut down and Harvey was airlifted to UCLA hospital where he spent the next two months in a coma. The helmet he was wearing surely saved his life.

Harvey had suffered a severe traumatic brain injury (TBI) along with many physical injuries, and he would spend the next six months in hospitals. From UCLA, he was transferred to Kindred Hospital in Culver City, and then to the Bakersfield Centre for Neuro Skills residential program.

It was in those first few weeks while Harvey was in a coma that his independence and civil rights would be terminated through a court-appointed conservatorship.

Harvey and his wife Sheila had been married for 16 years and had a six-year-old daughter. Having been born into privilege, Harvey had considerable wealth he had not co-mingled with his wife's accounts. Additionally, Harvey and Sheila had never prepared a will, power of attorney, or health care directive. Harvey felt he was a healthy 40-year-old, and he would handle those legal things when he was older.

Sheila and their daughter were living in their family home, where she was responsible for a hefty mortgage, even though she had limited access to Harvey's money. She hired an attorney and applied for conservatorship of Harvey and his assets. The case was heard by Judge Reva Goetz, who has handled such famous conservatorship cases as Britney Spears and Mickey Rooney.

Sheila was denied conservatorship over Harvey because they had recently separated and were living under different roofs. Even though she immediately rushed to his side in the hospital and resumed her role as his wife, the court decided they couldn't be certain whether or not Harvey would want Sheila to have continued access to his money.

Eventually Harvey's father and his attorney were awarded co-conservatorship and were able to pay general bills such as real estate and income taxes, utilities, groceries, etc. Harvey would eventually be awarded a monthly "allowance" to spend on whatever he wanted, making him feel like he was being treated like a child.

Once you've been put into a conservatorship, *you* can't hire an attorney, so one is appointed for you by the court. This attorney is called a Probate Volunteer Panel (PVP) attorney. Harvey's PVP attorney bragged at an initial meeting with Harvey and the family that she enjoyed causing friction between husbands and wives. She felt it was her duty to decide what was best for her client (Harvey) no matter what he or his family members might say to the contrary.

Harvey had a hearing every six months or so to monitor how things were going. He was supposed to be advised by his PVP attorney; however, she kept falsely telling the court Harvey wanted a continuance of the conservatorship. Harvey wanted his wife Sheila to be conservator, but the PVP attorney would not allow it, and argued for the continued humiliation of the court-monitored allowance for Harvey.

At the hearings, the lawyers—which by this point consisted of an attorney for his wife, an attorney for his father, Harvey's PVP attorney, and eventually a court-appointed attorney for his minor child (known as "guardian ad litem")—and the judge would talk about him as if he were a child (because basically without any of his rights, he sort of was). They would never refer to him by name, only as the "conservatoree." Harvey said it was very dehumanizing to be treated this way.

As Harvey began getting better and better, it was becoming obvious the conservatorship had to come to an end, but making that happen was harder done than said. He had to have a "capacity declaration" performed by a physician. The problem is when a large amount of money is at stake, doctors are reluctant to say yes, because if they said yes, and he lost it all the next day, the doctor's decision would be questioned.

Eventually Judge Goetz gave him the name of a specific doctor she trusted. Harvey would endure two days of rigorous testing, and in January 2011, the doctor eventually wrote a declaration that Harvey was responsible enough to control his own life. In March 2011 the judge terminated the conservatorship, and Harvey was once again granted all of his civil rights. After the hearing was over, the court reporter approached Harvey and told him she had sat in on thousands of cases like his, and his was only the third one she had ever seen terminated. It is *that* rare to have a conservatorship overturned.

However, Harvey's nightmare did not end there.

The court-appointed PVP attorney was supposed to charge at a reduced rate; however, she solicited the judge to bill at her full rate, and was granted permission. This frustrated Harvey, as he felt the lawyer really never had his best interests in mind. Harvey had to file for separate counsel to fight the fee petition, which added two more attorneys' fees. In addition to his PVP attorney's fees, he also received a bill from his father's attorney, the attorney who was acting as co-conservator, the guardian ad litem for his daughter, as well as his wife's attorney, despite the fact she had dropped her petition to be named conservator eighteen months prior. Harvey had to pay legal fees, bonding fees, and mandatory accounting fees.

In total, this cost him slightly over $1 million dollars, all because Harvey did not know he should have a durable power of attorney for health care and financial matters, and this created a situation where others took advantage of his health crisis.

Right after the conservatorship was lifted, Harvey told Sheila he wanted to go to Vegas and gamble... "because it was his money, dammit!" So in April 2011, Harvey wrote a holographic (handwritten) will in his own handwriting on a piece of paper that said, "Everything goes to my wife." Shortly afterward, he hired a law firm to implement all of their trusts, wills, power of attorney, etc.

Harvey wants everyone to understand the importance of having a durable power of attorney drawn up *now*, no matter your age or health because you never know when life takes a drastic turn like his did.

This durable power of attorney is a simple form you file with your attorney for a few hundred dollars, and it directs who is responsible for you and your estate, should you become incapacitated. Had he had one, it would have saved him the humiliation of losing his civil rights, as well as causing his loved ones time and grief, and of course, a million dollars in attorney and other fees.

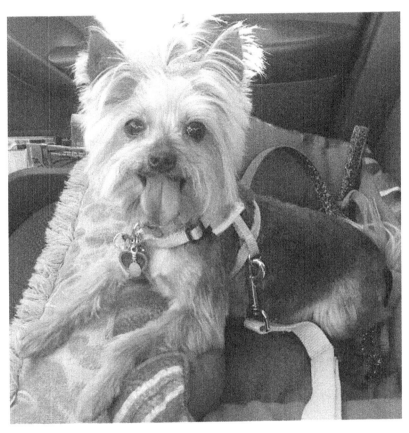

Pixxie is the best road-trip companion a gal could want.

Chapter Twelve

Who Rescued Whom? How My Yorkie Helped Me Cope After Brain Injury

May 2017

L ittle did I know when I initially rescued my Yorkie that she would end up rescuing me. The truth is, I had always been a "cat" woman. I had never owned a dog, and had heard how much work they are to take care of, so getting a dog wasn't ever on my radar.

I was recently divorced and feeling a little bit lonely, even though I had two cats at home, I still felt something was missing in my life. A woman who worked with me would bring her Chihuahua along to the photography studio on Wednesdays, and soon, I was thinking I could handle a little dog.

I reached out to the Carver-Scott Humane Society. A little Yorkie had come into the pound over the weekend. She had been abandoned by the side of the road, and was looking a little underweight and shabby. They warned me she wasn't very friendly, and would bare her teeth at anyone who tried to pick her up, but they were happy to bring her to my home for a meeting.

This lonely, scared little Yorkie showed up at my house and promptly peed in every section of the house (was she "marking her territory" because *she knew* she was staying?) When she finally let me pick her up—she licked my face and looked at me with her big brown eyes. It was pretty much puppy love at first sight.

Pixxie would go with me everywhere dogs were allowed. Friends thought of her more as my child than an actual dog, and even friends who weren't "dog people" would allow her to come to their home, and then say how sweet she was. At the Starbucks drive-thru her cuteness would command the attention of the entire staff, getting her very own "pupaccino" (mini cup of whipped cream.) She was also my new road-trip partner, traveling to 40 states and Canada, and truly my best friend.

Shortly after rescuing her, Pixxie and I moved to a new city where we both easily settled into our new loft. I was beginning to realize how much of a companion she truly was for me. Then on an Arctic-cold February morning, I fell on a patch of ice and landed full force on the back of my skull. Pixxie had been in my arms when I fell. Although she was quite shaken by what happened, she wasn't hurt. She was sitting about 10 feet from where I lay, looking at me with great "doggy concern," and for good reason. I had suffered a traumatic brain injury, along with whiplash and a dislocated sternum.

For the first several months I was completely dazed and confused, and would sleep for 12 to 14 hours at night. At first I was worried Pixxie would have a potty accident being in the bedroom during my long night's sleep, but she didn't. She knew I wasn't okay, and would give me extra snuggles and puppy kisses, and let me sleep in as late as I needed.

Pixxie could sense when I was in a lot of pain or was feeling depressed, and she would always come to my rescue, giving me reassuring licks after crawling up onto my lap. Even in my darkest days, she was by my side with those big ol' puppy eyes, letting me know she was there for me—even if I couldn't remember whether or not I had fed her dinner yet. She was my motivation to get up in the morning, and having a routine to take her out for her morning walk was a godsend.

I firmly believe having Pixxie kept me going when things got really hard. If I were frustrated or confused, sad or lonely, I would hear the sweet sounds of the little Yorkie I rescued only a year earlier. *It's truly hard to be sad when a dog is licking your face.*

Yes, I rescued Pixxie from a life of abandonment and mistreatment, but I believe she came into my life at just the right time to rescue me from an unexpected accident and period of darkness.

It's the proverbial cliché: who rescued whom?

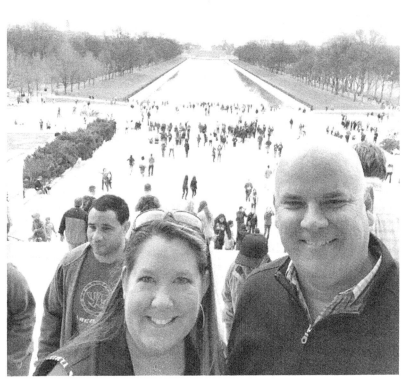

Hanging out with Paul in Washington, D.C. after
Congressional Brain Injury Awareness Day.

Chapter Thirteen

The Many Personalities of Brain Injury—
Why I Sometimes Want to Throw in
the Towel

June 2017

There is a saying in the brain injury community: "If you've seen one brain injury, you've seen one brain injury."

The premise of this saying is that no two brain injuries are the same, no two recoveries are the same, and no two treatment plans are the same. TBI is a complex and grossly misunderstood injury.

After sustaining a traumatic brain injury from a fall on the ice in February 2014, I have become an active advocate for the brain injury community. I have witnessed first hand the many ways TBI is misunderstood, and I have also witnessed the many different personality changes that can result from it.

Depending on where the brain has been injured, survivors can exhibit an array of behavioral and emotional symptoms including anger, rage, sensitivity, apathy, depression, lack of focus, loss of filtering, just to name a few.

I have noticed I am much more sensitive, and I am also more aware of the abusive behavior in other, seemingly well-meaning people.

As the administrator of a fairly large Facebook group for those with TBI, I have had my share of struggles in dealing with personal attacks from fellow brain injury survivors. Sometimes they lash out at me in frustration, anger, paranoia, and jealousy.

For the most part I understand that these attacks are their brain injury talking—and not really them, but knowing this certainly doesn't make it any easier to be on the receiving end of such attacks.

Sometimes I feel that the more visible I become in the brain injury community, the more I am punished by those who simply aren't able or don't understand how to control their behavior—and especially their words. It's a very real challenge, and I know I am not alone in being the brunt of these abusive attacks. Others who also are doing good work tell me that at times they, too, have been treated poorly.

One of the biggest obstacles I have to deal with is related to my first book, *Life With a Traumatic Brain Injury: Finding the Road Back to Normal,* which is a collection of my *HuffPost* pieces which shared my journey through the first 18 months of my recovery. I am often told I am working "to build an empire"—and trying to make money off the brain injury community.

Anyone who has ever published a book knows that the money we make from sales is "peanuts." The income I receive each month usually doesn't even pay my cell phone bill.

I get it. These people are struggling to make ends meet, and make assumptions I am rich because I am a published author. They feel I should be giving the money I earn back to the community, which I do indirectly. Every dollar I make on book sales, and through my GoFundMe page, is used to offset my travel costs for the advocacy work I am doing across the country.

But the reality is: I am barely making my own ends meet. I have come close to eviction because I couldn't come up with rent money in time. I have gone hungry for weeks at a time because I couldn't afford groceries. I have canceled meetings and appointments because I didn't have money to put gas in my car to get there. I have had my cell phone turned off on a fairly regular basis because I was late paying my bill. *That is my reality.*

I believe the readers of my articles often forget that I, too, am recovering from my own brain injury.

The reason I promote the heck out of my book is because I *know* it is helping those who read it—not because I am raking in cash from sales. Regularly, I hear from those who have read my book who tell me the stories saved their life, or helped them understand a loved one who is currently dealing with a brain injury. It's messages like these that keep me moving forward and keep me from getting too stressed out by the naysayer's comments and criticisms.

But with that said, the personal attacks still hurt.

I have become very comfortable with using the "block" button on Facebook, and do not hesitate to block anyone who is causing me stress. Some are far more relentless in their efforts, and will then do everything they can to find me online, seeking me out on Twitter, then LinkedIn, then my blog, and then email. It's sometimes scary, and I have at several points considered calling the police to see what my restraining options might be because one never knows if they will one day show up at my front door.

I have to say that even if a hundred people send me positive messages and only three send me negative, abusive messages, that three percent speaks the loudest. They are relentless at times, and drown out the positive messages I receive. I also understand this is partly my own processing (that may or may not have been affected by TBI), and I am taking action to work on overcoming my over-sensitivity.

But through it all, I *know* I am doing good by raising awareness of this invisible injury that affects 2.8 million Americans each year.

I have a vibrant, growing community on Facebook with many followers who are eager to help me spread my message. I have made many incredible friends in the brain injury world and *wouldn't trade this journey for anything.*

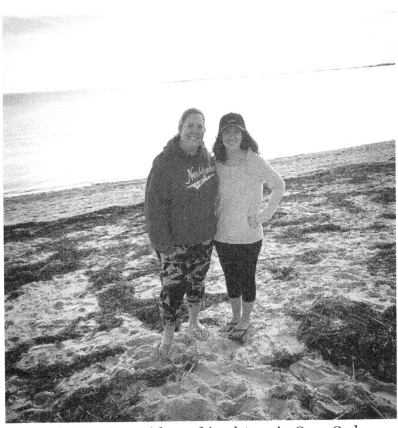

Enjoying time with my friend Amy in Cape Cod,
Massachusetts during a re-charge getaway.

Chapter Fourteen

Understanding Aphasia After
Brain Injury

June 2017

June is National Aphasia Awareness Month, and I wanted to share some of what I have learned on my journey through aphasia after brain injury.

According to Wikipedia, the term *aphasia* implies one or more communication modalities in the brain have been damaged—and are therefore functioning incorrectly. The difficulties for people with aphasia can range from occasional trouble finding words to losing the ability to speak, read, or write; however, their intelligence is un-affected.

Since no two brain injuries are ever the same, the way aphasia affects one person can vary greatly from the next person. In my own experience, I have had trouble finding the word I was expecting to come out of my mouth. I would be saying a sentence, and then all of a sudden, realize I had no idea what the word I was trying to say was supposed to be. It was the strangest feeling because the word simply vanished into thin air.

I also would say the wrong word, and not usually even realize it until the person I was talking to gave me a quizzical look. I would then ask him, "What did I just say?" For example, I had no idea I had said *flower* instead of *coffee pot.*

My reading and writing weren't affected by aphasia, but my cognitive processing of what other people were saying slowed greatly. I would sometimes not understand a word I knew I should know, and would have to ask them to tell me what it meant (which also would warrant quizzical looks).

It's such a strange experience because *you know you know* the word.

The biggest frustration I faced was when others around me would say something like, "Oh, I do that all the time, too," or "That's just part of getting older." (I wasn't even 40 at the time.) What others don't realize is this *isn't* something they are familiar with. I know what it was like pre-TBI to forget what you were trying to say or not know a word...typically it was an odd word you don't use often. But this is totally and completely different. You don't know it's not there until you go to say it, and then it doesn't come out.

I remember the very first time it happened to me. I was trying to tell a friend what I had seen on a billboard sign. I got to the word "billboard" and was so shocked that it didn't come out. I could describe what it looked like and what it said, but I simply couldn't come up with the word.

Richard from Minneapolis explains, "In 2003 I had a traumatic brain injury, and one of my main side-effects is, so to speak, aphasia. Because of aphasia, it's very easy for me to miss words or use the wrong words and perhaps, most importantly, not to understand what other people are saying."

In a recent podcast, I interviewed speech therapist, Rachel Katz. She talked about aphasia, which according to a study by Lam, J.M.C. & Wodchis, W. P. (2010), is most often the result of a traumatic brain injury or stroke, but doesn't affect intelligence, so it is not hard to understand the very real struggle of those experiencing it. In fact, a 2010 study involving more than 66,000 people about the impact of 60 different diseases and 15 conditions on quality of life found that aphasia has the largest negative impact on quality of life, more than cancer and Alzheimer's disease.

Katz went on to say, "Without the ability to communicate, your basic needs and wants aren't met." We all have word-finding difficulty at some point or another, but that is not necessarily aphasia. Aphasia is when it's beyond the norm. When you're looking at a cat, you know it's a cat, but you can't come up with the word cat. You say things like "It's furry and says meow!" to describe the word you're seeking.

Once you come up with that word and make the connection in your brain, you typically won't forget that word again, depending on the severity of your aphasia. You might be a little quicker to respond to the word next time. If you have a loved one with aphasia, you shouldn't always give her the word, but rather let her come up with it. If you continue to give her the word, and don't make her work through it, she has no motivation to work harder to get better.

> Mary from San Francisco, California said, "Aphasia and migraines are the remaining symptoms from my TBI from 2013. Aphasia is like playing the kids' game of describing something such as a zebra, but you can't use the most common words to describe it: black, white, striped, lives in Africa, looks like a horse."

My aphasia has greatly improved over the past three years of my recovery. I still find myself struggling for words when I am fatigued or stressed, but am impacted far less than the first 15 months of my journey.

There is always hope, and remember that just because you have word-finding problems, it does not mean you have diminished intelligence.

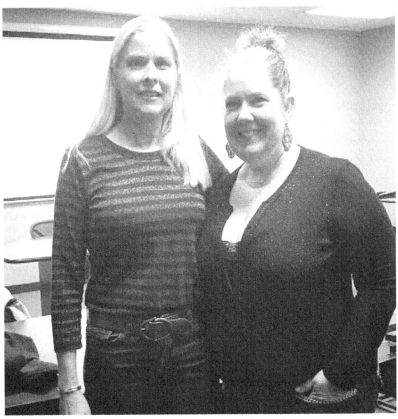

With Anne in Austin, Texas, attending the Brain Injury Alliance conference.

Chapter Fifteen

Living in a Funk: Depression and Apathy After Brain Injury

September 2017

D epression and apathy are symptoms of brain injury, and all too often are overlooked and dismissed by the medical community.

Before my brain injury, I don't recall suffering from depression or anxiety or sleeplessness—except for the occasional butterflies in my stomach before a big presentation, or not being able to sleep the night before an exciting big trip.

For the past two weeks I was in a deep, dark funk. I cried at the silliest things, I felt emotions swell up to the surface, and I had zero tolerance for others. I kept myself locked away in my house, not wanting to inflict my funk on anyone else. I avoided self-care and hygiene as it consumed too much energy, and apathy kept me paralyzed in place with a lack of motivation to get things done.

Casual acquaintances tell me, "Oh, that sounds like PMS," or "You must be peri-menopausal" or "It's just the moon cycle, I get like that too."

These comments drive me absolutely crazy.

I know *me* better than anyone, and I can tell you I have never experienced this prior to my brain injury. It's an all-too-common side-effect from hitting my head—scrambling the motherboard, so to speak.

I haven't felt this dark since the first year after my accident. The first year was filled with more days in a funk than not, but has since leveled off. So this particular episode of funk caught me off guard. I would start feeling better after a few days, and then slip back down into the hole of despair.

If you've never experienced it, it's super complicated and hard to comprehend.

People assume you should be able to "get yourself out of it" and shake it off, but it's truly not that easy. I am a positive person and know the exact steps you "should" take to bring yourself out of a funk, yet when I am in one, it's *so* freaking hard to do. Apathy (a neurologic problem that causes one to lack motivation) gets the best of me in times like these.

I'm pretty sure I know what tipped it off. I had traveled to Washington, D.C. to lobby for healthcare, followed by another trip to Columbus, Ohio, for the Concussion Health Summit where I spoke for three hours the first day, plus talked with a lot of other attendees and vendors.

I pushed myself too hard, and my body shut itself down in order to conserve energy.

In the early days after my injury, I wouldn't shower for days. You have no idea how much energy taking a shower and getting dressed takes, until you have limited supplies of it. It was such a daunting task, and I would *not* say this was depression—the issue was simply a lack of energy.

And that is exactly where I think medical professionals get it all wrong.

They write us off as depressed when in fact we are simply exhausted or over-stimulated. They don't understand that *apathy* is vastly different from depression. They try to put us on anti-depressants that *alter the chemicals in our brain,* which is trying to heal at that exact moment. Now, I am not saying meds are bad because some people truly need them. But in my case, I knew they weren't what my body needed, and I also knew they would hinder my recovery.

Now, I am three years out, and for the most part I have more good days than bad. I am feeling pretty good, even though I still need to nap, and have had to learn how to pace myself. However, when I have pushed myself, my body, and my brain too far, the funk returns.

I'll say this again because it bears repeating, the funk "depression" is a symptom of my brain injury. It doesn't mean I have mental health problems or that I'm unstable. It doesn't warrant medications that will make me feel worse. It requires rest, self-love, compassion, and maybe a box or two of chocolate.

When you notice a friend or loved one with a brain injury start to pull away and become disengaged, this is a sign they're in a funk.

Don't tell them to "get over it," or that they're being lazy. What they need is support and acceptance. Instead, give them a big hug and tell them how much you care about them. Ask how you can help, or better yet, jump in and help (laundry, cleaning, making meals, etc.). When we are in a funk, these tasks become way too much for us, and then they build up over time, making it that much more daunting.

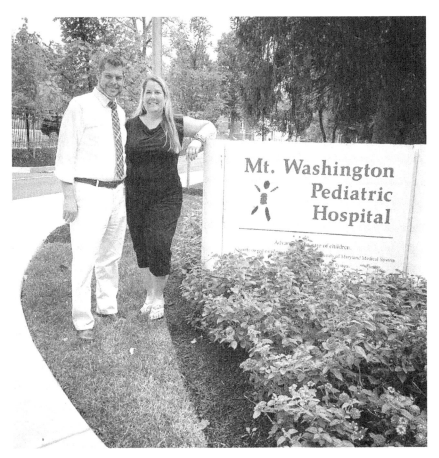

Spending time with Andy Wayne, Director of Marketing and Communications at Mt. Washington Pediatric Hospital.

Chapter Sixteen

Pediatric Hospital Creates Abilities Adventures Program for Brain Injury Patients

October 2017

As soon as you walk into Baltimore's Mt. Washington Pediatric Hospital (MWPH), you can tell it is unique. The building is full of an energy and a vibrancy that feels both welcoming and comforting.

Here you will find patients giggling in the hallways while doing rehab exercises with their therapists, allowing them to interact with staff and other patients who wander by. When asked what makes MWPH different, Chief Medical Officer, Dr. Richard Katz said, "The whole focus is towards the kids. There is no research or students, and the sole focus is on the care of these children. My favorite part of working here is the spirit of the employees; it's hard work but it's fun to come here."

Mt. Washington is a rehab specialty hospital that's a "step down" from acute, post-trauma, surgery or illness, and where the patients are now being prepared to return to their home life. In fiscal year 2017, they had 102 patient beds and admitted 700–800 patients, with *40 percent of in-patient admissions for children with brain injury* (traumatic, non-traumatic, and multi-trauma).

The focus of my visit is to meet the staff and learn about their "Abilities Adventures" trip to Utah, which provides the youth patients in their brain injury rehabilitation program to go on a 10-day adventure of a lifetime. The staff was preparing to leave on their second trip in a few weeks, and the excitement was buzzing.

Susan Dubroff runs the rehab program and is proud of their program because they follow their patients for five years past their exit from the hospital. *"Rehab doesn't stop when you leave the hospital, it continues and evolves.* This trip helps provide these patients with experiences— some have never been on a plane, and some have never been outside of Baltimore. By taking them to the National Abilities Center in Park City, Utah, they have access to the types of equipment they may need in order to participate in activities they never thought they could do," said Dubroff.

The whole concept of Abilities Adventures is to give patients life experiences and socialization, and help prove to them that they have the skills to do things which can change their lives. It also helps them understand there's more out there in the world, and gives them hope and a purpose.

Dubroff continued, "It's our responsibility to fully integrate someone back into their community. We help the patients understand they have the ability to do things they didn't think they would be able to do. We can give these kids exposure to things that help them build interests, strengths, and abilities."

Abilities Adventures is led by Lindie McDonough, who also specializes in helping patients reintegrate back into school. When she originally brought the idea of the trip to the board, she received some pushback due to safety concerns. They asked why not just do something locally, and she replied, "There are few resources for anyone with a brain trauma in the area, most of the adaptive sports cater to other disabilities. Additionally, the cost of doing a two-day, two-night trip locally costs as much as taking them for a full week to the National Abilities Center." The trip was funded by a grant from the Mt. Washington Pediatric Foundation Board, as well as supplemental funding from the National Abilities Center.

Dubroff added, "One of our strengths is dealing with brain injury. Our employees have an understanding of brain injury and have become involved with the local associations and pay attention to trends of how patients are getting their brain injuries."

Lindie expressed that seeing the kids learn how to advocate for themselves was amazing. Quite a few were in denial about their experiences of what happened to them or weren't comfortable asserting themselves in a way they need to. For instance, one girl was shivering because she was cold. When asked if she was cold she simply responded, "Yes." They had to prod her further to see if she needed a blanket, the heat turned up, or something else.

By the end of the trip she was speaking up, saying things like "May I please have another blanket."

The kids, as well as the parents, were quite nervous. Most of the kids had never flown, and were all at different stages of their recovery, but were ready to spread their wings and take some risks, even if they didn't know it yet.

Each evening, Lindie would email the parents with an update on what the kids did that day, including photos and videos. She also included some of her favorite quotes she overheard throughout the day from the kids—which showed how much fun they were having.

I had the opportunity to meet one of the participants, 14-year-old Ava, and her mother Ann. When I met Ava, I was greeted by her outgoing, sassy spirited personality, which I would learn was the result of going on the trip.

Ann told me her daughter, Ava, was zero percent nervous about going, while as her mom was 100 percent nervous. Ava had never been away from home since she first became sick in third grade. "They had all the parents and all the kids get together before the trip. Nothing is ever easy for these kids or for us. It was scary sending her so far away, but seeing her come back so confident was worth it!" The mom also said getting the emails at the end of each day was crazy—"I can't believe she's doing that!" was her typical response each night.

When I asked Ava why she wanted to go on this trip, she looked at me with a huge grin. "I was excited to get away from my parents and siblings!" She is hoping to become a peer mentor at the hospital, and her advice to any kids considering going on the trip was, "Just put your heart out there, and don't be scared to leave your parents."

Hearing Ava giggle and talk about the boys in her school leaves me completely awestruck that she was shy and introverted before the trip. The transformation in her confidence and personality is phenomenal, and is a typical transformation for the kids who go on these adventures.

Pediatric Neuropsychologist, Dr. Joseph Cleary, feels these trips are great at helping inspire these kids. "They may not be able to do what they did before their brain injury, but the trip helps them find a sense of joy and belonging."

Dr. Cleary believes it's all about creating the life you want, and figuring out a plan to get you there. "I have worked at a lot of places, and this is the smallest place I have ever worked, but has the biggest hearts. They really care, and you feel like you connect with patients. We give kids feedback on what they're really good at, because they're nervous about things they're not good at. We don't focus on the negatives, but, instead, use their strengths to help the child feel successful."

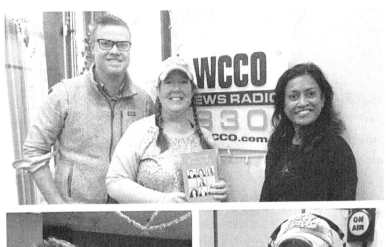

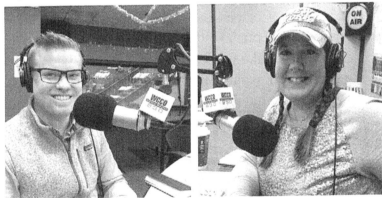

With Dr. Jeremy Schmoe and Roshini Rajkumar after completing our WCCO radio interview.

Chapter Seventeen

The Downside of Functional Neurology After Brain Injury

November 2017

When I slipped on the ice in February 2014, I truly had no idea the journey I was beginning—and how long it would take me to find a doctor who could help me with my 24/7 symptoms from a traumatic brain injury.

I would eventually spend two and a half years attending different doctor appointments as my full-time job, without getting answers or receiving the proper help I needed.

I began my journey by seeing a local chiropractor. Having been married to a chiropractor for almost 10 years, and understanding their very extensive education and skill level, I was much more comfortable seeing a chiropractor than a mainstream medical doctor.

Unfortunately, this chiropractor was only treating my physical symptoms (I had a slew of other physical injuries on top of the brain injury). I would constantly tell him I was dizzy and having trouble with my words, and my left eye seemed "off."

He would eventually send me to a neurologist, and this is where my frustration with the mainstream medical field would begin.

To start off on the wrong note, the neurologist was running 90 minutes late for my appointment. I'm not even entirely sure how it's possible to run that far behind, but it left me with approximately 15 minutes of her time, at the end of which she would tell me we need to give my brain injury "a little more time." If I wasn't feeling better *in six months,* I was to return for a re-assessment.

In six months I did return to the neurologist, still complaining of my short-term memory problems, dizzyness and balance issues, the deep fogginess inside my head I hadn't been able to shake, and the fact that my left eye still isn't feeling right. Once again, she didn't seem very concerned about my brain injury and told me to return in another six months—which now put me at *15 months out from my injury.* At this final appointment with her, she actually said, "Well, since it's a year out, this may be the best you're going to get."

WHAT?!

I cried. I begged for cognitive or occupational therapy—*anything* that could potentially improve my symptoms. *It was not acceptable that this was the best I would be* (and by this point I already knew about neuro-plasticity and the ability for the brain to recover). She eventually agreed to send me to Cranial Sacral Therapy (CST) and scheduled me for a neuropsychological exam to determine where my deficits were.

Long story short. The CST worked wonders to relieve the pressure in my head, but the neuropsych testing was a nightmare. Why hadn't the doctor sent me to this sooner?

The neuropsychologist basically told me I didn't try hard enough because I scored worse than a dementia patient in short-term memory (yet that was my biggest complaint). She suggested I be started on anti-depressants, Ritalin, and sleeping pills—all of which I politely refused, knowing they would only be a band-aid, and not actually help any of my symptoms.

Eighteen months after my accident I was feeling isolated, alone, and felt that doctors didn't believe me, so I began to accept that the way things were, was going to be my new normal. For the next year I moved through life feeling like I was constantly swaying on a boat, and I would regularly bump into door jams, I couldn't read more than a few pages of a book at a time (when I used to be an avid reader), and my short-term memory was pretty much non-existent (making running my own business quite a challenge).

Enter Dr. Schmoe

At the two and a half-year mark, I received a message from Dr. Schmoe at Minnesota Functional Neurology DC. He had read one of my *HuffPost* pieces—and told me he could help me. By this point I had already given up on doctors, and wasn't interested in yet another doctor who would soon tell me he can't help me.

I finally relented and told myself "what could it possibly hurt?" As I said in earlier articles, I am so glad I decided to go in for a consultation.

Dr. Schmoe spent *two hours* with me in his initial consult, testing my eyes, balance, cognitive abilities, and so much more. He confirmed my eyes indeed weren't tracking together properly, which is why my left eye had "felt off." It was also why I was experiencing constant dizziness and balance problems. He worked with me over the course of two weeks, with *90-minute therapy appointments* focusing on eye and head movements, incorporated with both full-body movements and hand-eye coordination exercises.

I noticed almost immediate relief. My dizziness and balance issues were nearly 100 percent gone. My mental clarity felt clearer, and I was finally able to improve my short-term memory. Gradually over the next few months I would feel that other symptoms, such as over-stimulation and extreme fatigue, were slowly slipping away.

Now, don't get me wrong. My symptoms aren't 100 percent gone. I still have flare-ups, and if I overdo things, I will set myself back. But I went from feeling only 50 percent myself to 90 percent myself. I now know how to do the exercises wherever I am in order to calm the symptoms back down if I have a flare-up.

The Downside of Functional Neurology

There is a downside to functional neurology—not a single doctor referred me to functional neurology, and I had never heard of it before Dr. Schmoe reached out to me. Because it's not a mainstream medical profession, folks are skeptical of it—even though mainstream doctors haven't been able to help them.

I have actually received attacks and hate mail for my loud-and-proud stance on functional neurology. I have been accused of receiving kickbacks (payment for patient referrals)—which is a bold accusation since it is completely illegal across all healthcare professions. I have been yelled at because many don't accept insurance. I have been lectured on how a chiropractor or functional neurologist shouldn't be allowed to touch anyone with a brain injury. I have been belittled and told functional neurology is a sleazy, snake-oil scam, and everyone should be made aware of their gimmicks.

Here's the thing. Every single medical profession has its fair share of bad apples. As you've gathered from this article, I was less than thrilled with my neurologist (whom I am convinced received her diploma from a Cracker Jack box) and the neuropsychologist should have her credentials taken away for the way she treated me. I have been to chiropractors and MDs who I am amazed have managed to receive their degree.

My point is: if you don't like a particular doctor, that's fine. If you've had a bad experience, it's okay to talk about it. It's always okay to "fire" your doctor if they aren't listening to you. But it is *not* fair to bash an entire healthcare profession because of "something you read on the internet," or because of something someone you know only through Facebook told you.

I remember how much it hurt when people would say to me about my chiropractor husband, "Oh, so he's not a *real* doctor."

Functional neurology helped me when all other doctors and professionals had let me down.

I had given up on my recovery, which is a very scary place to be. I will never stop talking about functional neurology because it's not fair to the other millions of TBI survivors who are still struggling and have never heard of it.

With that said, not all functional neurologists specialize in brain injury and concussion, therefore, you do need to do your research. If you're not sure where to start, give Minnesota Functional Neurology DC a call and they will gladly help you find someone near you.

Functional neurology uses specifically designed therapies to enhance the performance of your brain and nervous system. This unique approach offers new hope for people suffering from a wide variety of conditions. Most functional neurologists have 1500-plus hours of education beyond chiropractic school specifically on the nervous system, and will spend hours instead of minutes with you at each appointment. They take a functional approach to each individual patient, and create a very specific treatment plan unique to the patient's symptoms.

Functional neurology gave me back a quality of life I thought I was never going to find again, and for that I am forever grateful.

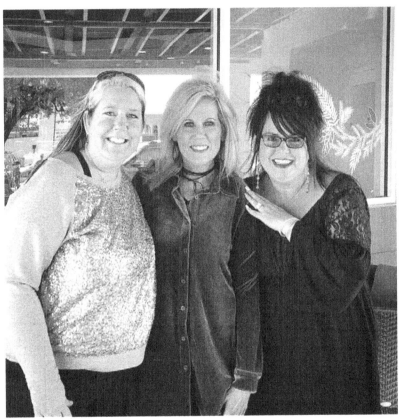

Meeting Cyndy and Shelley in Dallas, Texas.

Chapter Eighteen

Six Tips For Surviving the Holidays and Overstimulation With a TBI

December 2017

With the holidays upon us, many traumatic brain injury (TBI) survivors will find themselves facing more overstimulation than normal, which can cause additional brain fatigue and stress, as well as causing fear and panic to set in for some situations.

Overstimulation is one of the most common symptoms among TBI patients, and can come in any combination of sounds, images, light, smell, taste, and touch.

Because overstimulation can't be "seen," it can be a mystery to those who have never experienced it, and can cause frustration between someone going through it and their loved ones who don't understand it.

Personally, I have a hard time dealing with a crowded restaurant or mall this time of year because there is too much noise that's combined with lights and lots of scents. I will have a hard time focusing when there is a lot of background noise, and find myself unable to carry on a conversation or make sense of what I am trying to do. I will leave feeling completely exhausted and often acquire a headache to go with it. I usually tire out before my 80-year-old mother, who can shop circles around me.

I have compiled a list of six simple things you can do to make the holidays easier on yourself or a loved one who is dealing with overstimulation.

1. **Keep hydrated.** The brain functions best when it is fully hydrated. When you are out shopping, it is easy to become dehydrated rather quickly. You can combat this by always having a water bottle with you and refilling it often. As tempting as it is, drinking alcohol and caffeine will also cause you to get dehydrated, so it is best to avoid those types of drinks when you know you are going to be faced with overstimulation.

2. **Keep additional stimulation to a minimum.** Decrease the amount of stimulation in places where you have control. If you know you're headed to the mall or a crowded restaurant, don't watch television before heading out or listen to the radio on the way there. If you're going with a friend or loved one, explain to them you might not be able to have a conversation while you're there. Bring your sunglasses and earplugs, and use them if you need them.

3. **Get additional rest.** While this one seems obvious, it is sometimes hard to do with the hustle and bustle of the holiday season. Rest is critical to helping our brain recover from overstimulation. Take a nap before or after your big outings, and do your best to get a good night's sleep each night. Give

yourself a designated bedtime, and stick with that schedule throughout the holidays.

4. **Take shorter trips.** If you have a lot to get done, you may want to consider breaking it up into smaller trips. I find it easier to do one errand each day, rather than trying to cram five things into one outing. It may take longer, but your brain will thank you.

5. **Write lists.** I am the queen of sticky notes and shopping lists. Don't add additional stress to the situation by going shopping without a clear list of where you need to go and what you need to get. Even with a list, it is easy to feel overwhelmed and out of sorts. Having a plan of exactly where you need to go, and what you need to purchase at each location, will help keep your stress levels down and keep you organized.

6. **Ask for help.** It can be hard to do, but sometimes you need to ask for help, whether it's asking someone to drive you somewhere, carry your bags, or even run an errand for you. Know when you've reached your limits (or, preferably *before* you've reached your limits) and ask for help. If you're a friend or loved one, offer help before it's asked for, or better yet, go ahead and do something that's on their list before you see they need assistance.

If you are a caregiver, family member, or friend of a TBI survivor, please understand that overstimulation is very real. Allow us to take the steps needed to ensure our health and sanity this holiday season and all year round.

To all my fellow TBI survivors, take care of yourself, and give yourself grace when needed. It is easy to push ourselves because we feel like we have so much to get done; however, it is important to know when to step back...and take a nap.

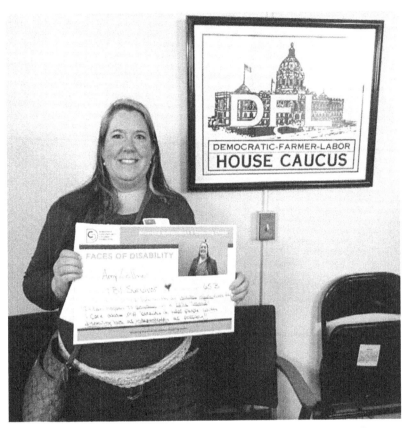

Advocating at the Minnesota State Capitol with the
Minnesota Brain Injury Alliance.

Chapter Nineteen

It's Not Like You Have Cancer
or Something

January 2018

When sharing my concussion diagnosis, someone I thought was a friend actually wrote these words on social media, "It's not like you have cancer or something." They cut deeper than a knife, and have wounded me for nearly the four entire years since my fall.

This is a story I have kept bottled up inside, unsure of how to express myself without sounding like a whiny brat. She was right; I *didn't* have cancer. But her dismissal of my concussion on social media—and the "likes" it received from others who I also thought were friends—absolutely devastated me. It caused me to clam up and not talk at all about my accident or my recovery for an entire year.

And still, it took facing a cancer diagnosis for me to finally understand the depths of her accusations.

Because, she wasn't right at all.

Last fall, my mother was diagnosed with breast cancer. I will preclude this story with the fact it was caught early, was very small, with less than 12 percent chance of recurrence, and she is doing great.

It's not the call you ever want to receive from your mother (or anyone), but I am eternally grateful for this experience. What happened with my mom's journey taught me a lot about the utter and complete lack of understanding by friends, families, and healthcare professionals when it comes to concussion and brain injury.

As soon as my mom's mammogram looked suspicious, they scheduled a biopsy, which came back as cancerous. She was whisked away to the oncologist and surgeon who prepared her and my father for what to expect over the next several months. She would have a lumpectomy to remove the tumor, followed by five weeks of daily radiation therapy.

What I witnessed next was wonderful.

Her friends were *amazing*. They rallied around her with support and encouragement, offering to help in any way they could, whether she needed rides, meals, or companionship. My dad was tremendous and stepped up as best he could to be her rock.

This is a stark contrast to what I experienced in the days, weeks, and months following my own fall on the ice that created an extreme medical crisis. Friends drifted away. Doctors didn't know how to help me. My family didn't understand the scope of my pain, frustration, and depression. When I shared my diagnosis, I was ridiculed by a lot of people who I thought were actual friends, who told me to quit feeling sorry for myself because it's not like I had cancer or something.

It still pains me deeply to remember.

I could choose to wallow in self-pity—or to use my pain to help others by making something beautiful from a dark situation. This is why I turned to writing as a way to not only help myself sift through the layers of emotions, but also to help others on a similar journey make sense of this crazy double standard.

Whatever it is that each of us is going through, whether it's a medical condition, a loss of a loved one, financial difficulty, illness, or *anything* you deem as a "big deal," you have every right to express your feelings.

Nobody else has the right to tell you that whatever it is you're experiencing isn't "bad enough." Yes, someone is always going to have it worse, and is going through something bigger. But that doesn't mean it's not okay for you to ask for help when you need it, or even have some self-pity.

Whatever is a big deal in our own life is a *big deal*. My mother's cancer diagnosis was a big deal for me, even though it wasn't *me* who had cancer. Yes, my concussion was a *big deal* to me because I couldn't even figure out how to use the microwave or remember what day of the week it was. I was living with a hell inside my head that nobody else could see or understand.

I am thankful for the former friend who ridiculed me, for without her ignorant and frustratingly awful words, I may never have written my first piece for *HuffPost*. While

I terribly miss my group of former friends, their true colors have shown me what so many other TBI survivors face every single day: there is a total and complete lack of understanding of this invisible injury that affects over 2.8 million Americans each year.

Advocate for Yourself

My advice to anyone on this journey who is feeling isolated and misunderstood is to find a local support group. Getting out, even once a month, and interacting with other folks who have similar experiences can be amazingly helpful. If you don't have the means to do that, find an online group such as my Tribe on Facebook.

Check out my "suggested reading" list for books that can help you understand this crazy journey you're on, and it will help friends and family understand.

Also, reach out to your state Brain Injury Association or Alliance and see if they have any further resources. They typically have activities throughout the year where you can participate or volunteer.

Lastly, you are always welcome to call the Brain Injury Association of America's 800 number. They will do their best to help you find local resources: 1-800-444-6443.

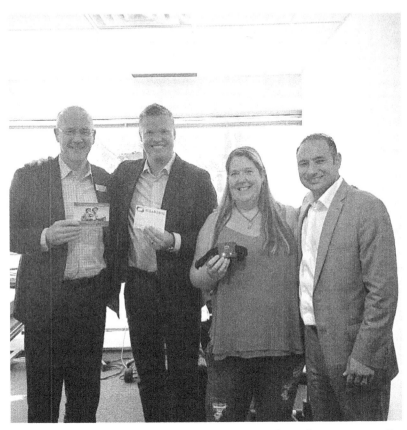

Dr. Jeremy Schmoe and I meeting with Mike Horn and Chrys Chrysanthou from ClearEdge.

Chapter Twenty

Former Wall Street Exec Turns Focus to Concussion and Brain Health

January 2018

Rich Uhlig was happily retired from Wall Street and enjoying his son's hockey game when the unexpected happened—his son took a hard hit into the boards. As everyone scrambled to make sure he was okay, Rich wondered if his son had received a concussion. No one could give him a definitive answer, which made him begin to ponder: how we can carry a phone in our pocket that can tell us just about anything we need to know, yet no one can determine if his son suffered a concussion.

"I'm a naturally curious person," Rich stated, which is what led him to begin looking into concussion research. He was shocked at how little there was out there to help athletes and coaches determine whether someone had a concussion, and what did exist was too subjective for his liking—the market needed an objective tool.

This would lead Rich out of retirement to begin a research company of his own that would dig deeper into concussions and begin working on a device to be used to track changes in an athlete's balance and reaction time. He would also begin studying saliva and its connection to being able to *not only detect concussion,* but also determine how long *it will likely take the person to recover.*

Rich joked, "I'm easily bored," when I asked him how difficult was the decision to leave retirement and go back to working long hours. His passion to help prevent concussions, and to help those struggling with lingering symptoms get the help they need, is evident. "I'm doing all of this for my son," he added.

"I'm one of those people who love a challenge and love to learn, so diving head-first into this (sorry about the pun!) was just part of who I am. At this point, I feel like everything I've done previously was just a prelude and training ground to prepare me for the triumphs and struggles associated with building what is now Quadrant Biosciences. Realizing early on that our work had the potential to improve the lives of so many children and adults certainly added a sense of urgency to our mission," Rich said.

It began with an idea of putting a device into helmets to track concussive hits, but he quickly knew it wouldn't provide the answers. "Collisions can't provide an objective diagnosis," Rich said.

He knew they wanted to provide physicians with the best tools to acquire the data necessary to make objective decisions, and also to make it patient-friendly so they can access their data from anywhere in the world. For instance, if an athlete switched schools or states, his or her data would be easily available to a new physician.

146

In March 2012, Rich self-funded Motion Intelligence, which would later become Quadrant Biosciences. In 2013, Quadrant had connected with SUNY Upstate Medical University, and in 2015 moved its office onto campus in the Institute for Human Performance building.

Collaborating with the Upstate Concussion Clinic, Motion Laboratory, Neuroscience, and the Molecular Analysis Core Facility at SUNY, Rich and his team created a product called ClearEdge. ClearEdge includes FDA-cleared computerized tests and a cloud-based system for storage and retrieval of the test results, and it was launched for sale in August 2017.

The ClearEdge Brain Health Toolkit *provides* a new standard of care that offers clinical best practices with cloud-based analytics. The ClearEdge Toolkit offers clinicians a suite of testing applications that have the following desirable characteristics:

- **Complete** — ClearEdge provides clinicians a suite of tests and assessments to establish baselines and track brain health and wellness over time. The toolkit is comprised of separate tests for cognitive efficiency, balance assessment, and symptoms tracking.
- **Objective** — Patient test results are quantitatively analyzed relative to prior performance.
- **Reliability** — The test-retest reliability of the cognitive and balance tests enable clinicians to identify

changes in a patient's performance that exceed the normal range of variability.

- **Evolutionary** — Academic research is translated to clinical practice.
- **Cost-Effective** — The system's low cost of acquisition and short testing interval (approximately 20 minutes) facilitates time-and-revenue efficiencies using existing CPT codes.
- **Portable** — The entire system fits in a briefcase; ClearEdge testing can be done almost anywhere.

Additionally, Rich's team has also focused a lot of effort on developing a saliva test that may be used in the future to detect a concussion.

There has been a big push by researchers to find a reliable biomarker test to objectively diagnose a concussion, but thus far it has remained elusive. However, the research Quadrant is conducting in cooperation with Penn State College of Medicine and SUNY Upstate Medical University may change that. Focusing on sampling patients' saliva, a set of micro RNAs have been identified that are present in significantly different amounts in patients with a con-cussion versus normal patients. Among the significant findings of this research include:

- **Saliva, a Rich Source** – MicroRNAs have been found in relative abundance in the saliva which, when coupled with their unique epigenetic properties, make them attractive biomarker candidates.

- **Accurate Differentiation** – Six microRNAs had parallel changes in CSF and saliva, and could accurately separate concussion and control cases.
- **Predictive of Symptom Duration** – The study also showed compelling data that this biomarker may be a better predictor of symptom (headache, fatigue, difficulty concentrating, etc.) duration than current standard concussion assessments.

Results of this research were presented at the 2017 Pediatric Academic Societies meeting in San Francisco, and published in the highly regarded medical journal, *JAMA Pediatrics*.

I was fortunate to meet Rich and his team in Syracuse, New York, after Motion Intelligence President, Chrys Chrysanthou, reached out to me after reading my story on *HuffPost*, and introduced me to the research and development that Quadrant were doing.

When I sat down with Rich, I was immediately drawn to his passion to find a solution—which rivaled my own passion for advocacy. He told me, "I see us making a difference. If we do that, then we've done it right!"

Rich and his team are dedicated to finding objective solutions, and strive to meet the gold standard of quality. The entire team is passionate about finding answers and providing tools that will help diagnose and give patients a sense of understanding. He started this journey out of an effort to help his son, but every other individual who sustains a concussion will benefit from his passion.

He concluded by stating, "Quadrant Biosciences is an incredible group of people from very diverse backgrounds. Every day, I'm humbled by their intellect and ability to innovate. I'm old enough to know how special this company is, and what a privilege it is to work with everyone here!"

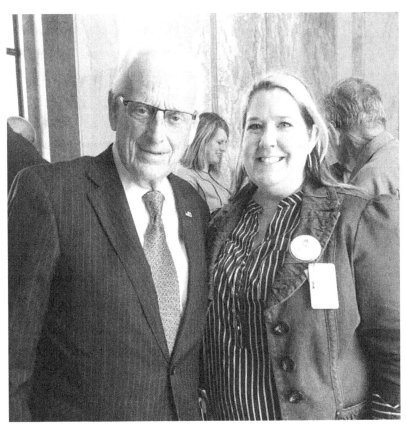

Working with Congressman Pascrell (NJ), who founded
the Congressional Brain Injury Task Force in 2001.

Chapter Twenty-one

How Minnesota Is Helping to Solve the Concussion Epidemic Through Research and Innovation

January 2018

While Minneapolis is preparing to host Super Bowl 2018 in a few short weeks, Twin Cities' researchers are coming together to present their innovations to the public in an array of events.

It seems fitting that as Minnesota gears up to host the biggest game in football, it would highlight some of the most advanced thinking and innovations around concussions. *What makes the Twin Cities so robust* is a three-fold combination of 1) high-quality academics, 2) financial support and funding for research, and 3) a large med-tech community.

With football being at the center of attention in the concussion debate, it only seems appropriate Minnesota would take this opportunity to shed light on all of the groundbreaking work being done in the state.

I had the pleasure of interviewing several of the acclaimed innovators who will be featured during the week leading up to Super Bowl 2018. These series of events around the Twin Cities are open to the public (most are free). They are designed to give us a glimpse into the amazing work geared toward the advancement of concussion prevention and treatment that's occurring right in our own backyard.

Whether you're a football fan or not, you will be enlightened by this lineup of incredibly smart and talented Minnesotans.

The Events

January 19 *Impact on the Gridiron: Safety, Accountability, and the Future of Football*

This event is not about undermining the game of football, or any other contact sport, for that matter. Instead, it's designed to tackle key issues facing players, teams, leagues, doctors and lawyers regarding head injuries and brain trauma. Leading experts share perspectives on medical advances in the diagnosis and treatment of chronic traumatic encephalopathy (CTE), related legal and ethical issues, youth athletics and parental concerns, player representation, and the sports fan's appetite for football in light of concussions.

January 30 *Startup Capital of the North Showcase*

This event is designed to showcase the breadth of innovation across the Startup Capital of the North, including the rapidly growing sports-tech community. Hear from the founders of an all-star lineup of MN Cup winners over the past decade, followed by an hour of demonstrations given by emerging local sports and student startups.

January 31 *Minnesota Spinal Cord and Traumatic Brain Injury Research Symposium*
This event is near and dear to me. I had lobbied with the Minnesota Brain Injury Alliance during the Legislative session at the State Capitol every Tuesday this past year. We were part of a grassroots advocacy effort led by Get Up Stand Up To Cure Paralysis (GUSU). We were successful in our efforts to get the Spinal Cord and TBI research grant funded with $6 million for the next biennium (2 years). "This was a major grassroots victory for spinal cord and brain injury advocates, and clearly demonstrates what is possible when funding is made a priority in the minds of state legislators," commented Jeff Nachbar, Public Policy Director of the Minnesota Brain Injury Alliance. During this half-day symposium moderated by Dr. Uzma Samadani, MD, PhD, and Walter Low, PhD, participants will hear from researchers whose innovative projects have been funded by this grant, as well as the progress of their projects.

February 1 *Player's Health Super Bowl Summit*
Moderated by KARE 11's Tim McNiff, Francis Shen from the Neurolaw Lab, and Troy Pearson, director of the Timberwolves and Lynx Basketball Academy. The Player's Health Summit is focused on gathering professional athletes, sports medicine professionals, leaders in sports administration, risk management professionals, and coaches, to explore best practices of health and safety in youth sports today and in the future.

February 2 *SportCon*

Explore the many ways in which data-driven decision-making continues to play a major role in sports, with a stellar lineup of speakers from academia, professional teams and the tech industry. In addition to individual technical and business-oriented talks, the conference will feature panels on data in fantasy sports, sports tech, and collegiate analytics, and more, plus a "Startup Showcase" session, in which up to 10 promising sports-tech startups will each do a six-minute pitch. This free event is perfect for sports fans, as well as analytics enthusiasts from any field.

The Innovators
Brain Injury Research Lab

Located in Hennepin County Medical Center (HCMC), which is the largest level-one trauma center in the state of Minnesota and one of the busiest in the United States, the lab is led by Dr. Uzma Samadani, MD PhD, neurosurgeon and brain injury researcher. She serves as the Rockswold Kaplan Endowed Chair for Traumatic Brain Injury at HCMC and as an Associate Professor of Neurosurgery at the University of Minnesota. She is also an attending neurosurgeon at the Minneapolis Veterans Administration Medical Center.

The Brain Injury Research Lab is using innovative technology that measures eye movement to better detect and classify concussions and other brain injuries that are invisible to radiological scans such as CTs and MRIs. This technology has the potential to revolutionize the assessment of brain function in real time.

Samadani said, "The reality is one person could have multiple symptoms from a single concussion, while another person has no symptoms even after multiple concussions. These things are so complicated—and not as straightforward as we would like to believe. We believe that eye-tracking will be a very important component in classifying, treating, and preventing brain injury."

In addition to eye-tracking, the research lab is also working with the team at Iron Neck to determine the role that neck strength plays in preventing concussions, particularly in women. "For women it is definitely more of a problem. We have longer, thinner necks and are like a bobblehead. I don't think we realize how vulnerable we are. I can see how any impact to the body could potentially create more of a jostle in women than men because they don't have the same core strength in the neck," Samdani stated.

The lab is also working on several other projects, includeing saliva testing, Vagus Nerve stimulation, blast injuries, and the Minnesota Healthy Brain Initiative.

Shen Neurolaw Lab

Led by Dr. Francis Shen at the University of Minnesota, the Neurolaw Lab is translating advances in brain science into better law and policy.

In the emerging field of neuroscience and law, the basic idea is that there are laws governing human brain (ex: auto accidents), and the more that is understood about how the human brain works, a better job can be done to create policies and laws to protect our brains. Shen said, "The big challenge is trying to determine what, if anything, in science advances, but not enough to give you a clear answer. Clinicians have these same challenges; however, in law judges have to decide whether to admit evidence into a trial, or how much money to award in damages."

According to Dr. Shen, "There is a great interest in continuing to promote concussion awareness and education, but at the same time there is an awareness that providing information simply isn't enough. Athletes, coaches, and parents are learning more but the evidence isn't clear enough as to whether we are seeing enough changes in practice. We need more data and more objective methods for defining and detecting concussions." He added, "We need better measures and data of concussions, and not just wait until symptoms show up."

Shen also noted that currently all grades K-12 have a "return to play" law, yet less than half the athletes and parents know about the law, which has existed since 2012.

Prevent Biometrics

Steve Washburn, CEO and co-founder David Sigel, Chief Marketing Officer. Developed over 6 years ago in collaboration with neurosurgeons and engineers at the

Cleveland Clinic, and then established in Minneapolis in 2015, Prevent Biometrics' patented technology is the first and only real-time concussion-impact monitoring technology.

Embedded in a mouth guard and paired with a mobile app, Prevent Biometrics' head-impact monitor continuously monitors the athlete, and records every head impact received. If an impact exceeds a preset threshold, a red LED light immediately illuminates on the mouth guard and an alert is sent to personnel on the sidelines through the mobile app. This app not only shows the athlete's impact history, but also the force, location, and direction of the impacts; thus collecting crucial data for future research.

With a plus-or-minus-five margin of error, it is the only product to meet the NFL's validation standard for head impact. Sigel said, "Helmet systems tend to be very inaccurate, as the helmet can move independently of the head. A mouth guard is held rightly in place by your teeth; when your teeth/jaw move, your head also moves."

Sigel also stated that they are not *preventing* concussions; they are trying to find undetected concussions. Over 50 percent of concussions go undetected, undiagnosed and untreated, which can lead to severe neurological problems. Their device allows coaches, trainers, and sideline personnel to make a more accurate, data-informed decision about whether the athlete needs to be assessed for concussion.

Players Health

Founder Tyrre Burks knows first-hand the reality of sports injuries. Having played sports throughout his childhood, and several years on the Canadian Football League, led him to develop a risk-management application to help sports organizations track their player's injuries and health, and to remain compliant with the state's safety protocols.

Launched in July of 2016, Burks' application already has over 90,000 users, including coaches, parents, administrators, athletic trainers, as well as the athlete. When Burks began research looking into sports organizations, he found that most were operating with safety guidelines that were 10 or more years outdated. He found the information wasn't being communicated properly, and there was no way to monitor the new guidelines because no one was policing it.

He also found that in 90 percent of the local club-level sports, no athletic trainer is at the practice. With parents paying thousands of dollars for their child to play in a club, priority should be to have an athletic trainer at the game.

Burks said, "The recreation program is now seeing a huge decline in numbers because of the club market. As a parent, you need to be concerned about the safety of your child, not how fancy the jerseys are."

TackleBar Football

Founded by football parents, Jeremy and Brigid Ling, TackleBar has launched a safer approach to football that preserves the traditions and fundamentals of the game, while reducing the risk of concussions and other injuries associated with tackling. Their mission is to dramatically reduce both head injuries and all other injuries related to tackling, while at the same time preserving the spirit of the game.

Wearing traditional helmet, shoulder pads, and a patented TackleBar harness around their torso, the ball carrier is downed by tearing off one of the bars. The design teaches proper defensive fundamentals as the bar location requires the defense to play with their head up and eyes on the ball carrier at all times.

TackleBar's CEO, Tim Healy, said, "We have been around football our whole lives, and some of the greatest life lessons we've learned and relationships we've built have stemmed from this game. This is an innovative change to the game at a time when we need to make the game safer and more appealing to both youth and parents."

MinneAnalytics

MinneAnalytics is a nonprofit organization dedicated to serving Minnesota's data science and analytics community. They are the largest regional community and events organization in the U.S.

They facilitate sharing knowledge and ideas among analytics professionals across business, technology and decision science through their industry-specific events and conferences. In addition, they host student analytics challenges, analytics leader forums, and provide student scholarships. MinneAnalytics' events are free to attend because of sponsor's gracious help.

"We expect at least 1,000 participants to attend SportCon based on the huge success of last year's event," said Dan Atkins, co-founder and executive director of MinneAnalytics. "It drew a wide array of experts, analysts, and thought leaders from all parts of the sports world— and that included management personnel from every one of our Minnesota professional sports teams."

Their community has grown to more than 11,500 members. This highly educated and well-placed mix includes professionals with job titles ranging from CEO to Quantitative Analyst. The variety of organizations ranges from the Fortune 500, to startups, academia, and the curious.

Ben Utecht

Ben Utecht is best known for his role as Super Bowl champion tight end for the Indianapolis Colts, playing alongside quarterback Peyton Manning. In addition to his football career, he is also a gifted musician, author, motivational speaker, and loving husband and dedicated father to four beautiful girls.

Utecht told me that at its core, his book is a memoir, an opportunity for him to chronicle his football story, as well as the story of meeting his wife and the births of his daughters—so he has a way to tell his daughters about it, in case one day he no longer remembers any of it.

"I am not a bitter man, I love football. I want to see it done the right way, at all levels. I want to tell a story that makes people consider, for the first time maybe, how critical their mind is to their identity. If that shifts as a culture, it will have a great impact on the brain health of athletes," said Utecht.

His message to parents is simple:

1. Educate yourself fully, understand what a concussion injury and its symptoms are, and what to do if it happens to your child.
2. If you want your children to play sports, build a relationship with a neurologist and get a baseline assessment of your child.
3. Understand that between the ages of 2—12 is when your child's brain is going through the most growth and developmental changes. Don't enter your child into sports until after age 12.

Utecht hopes sharing his story will help spread a message on the importance of our memory and brain health. Speaking and giving leadership programs have become his passion, saying, "Speaking is about influencing just one. It's not about how many people you're in front of, it's the impact your words can have, even if it's just one person—because that one person could turn your message into something for millions. You never know when you're going to be the miracle for somebody."

Minnesota Functional Neurology, DC

Dr. Jeremy Schmoe at Minnesota Functional Neurology DC (MFNC) is paving the way in Minnesota with his progressive approach to concussion recovery. His clinic is staffed with a team of caring and dedicated practitioners integrating neuroscience clinically.

Dr. Schmoe has developed a weeklong intensive program in which he and his team see a patient for three one-hour rehab sessions per day for a five-day period. He has found that this approach has decreased symptom severity in chronic post-concussion patients. He has patients travel from all across the country to work with him.

MFNC is equipped with cutting-edge diagnostic tools and rehabilitation equipment including: Ocular-Motor Graphing Software, Dynavision D2, Platform Posture Analysis, Video Gait Analysis, Clear Edge Brain Health Baseline, Low-Level Laser Therapy, ARPwave Neuro-Therapy, Non-Invasive Nerve Stimulation, Chiropractic Manual Therapy, Functional Blood Chemistry Analysis and Functional Neuro-Orthopedic Rehabilitation.

"I see patients who have been told there is *no hope for recovery*. For me, that is just not good enough. If there is *any* ability to build plasticity and change the brain, I am going to find it and attempt to make improvements. I never give up on patients, and I enjoy being the provider who offers them hope. I have seen some amazing things happen in our clinic, and to many people, they seem like miracles. It is common for us to see these improvements when the brain is given the *appropriate stimulation and environment to heal.* There's nothing better than hearing that we helped change a patient's life—or got him or her back doing the activities they love to do," said Dr. Schmoe.

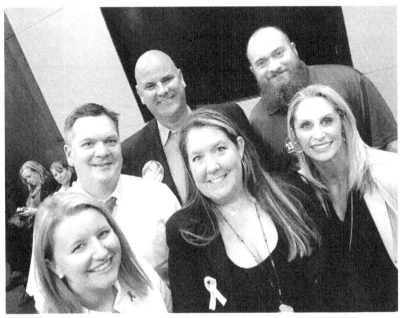

With a few of my fellow Brain Injury Advisory Council members in Washington, D.C. for Congressional Brain Injury Awareness Day: Sarah, Greg, Paul, Josh, and Stephanie.

Chapter Twenty-Two

Spotlights: Brain Injury Advisory Council Members

Anne Forrest, Ph. D.

Anne Forrest is an original member of the Brain Injury Association of America (BIAA) Brain Injury Advisory Council (BIAC), which was established by BIAA President and CEO Susan Connors in 2008 to provide input and feedback on a broad range of activities, especially those involving brain injury awareness and advocacy.

Anne sustained a traumatic brain injury (TBI) in 1997 when she was rear-ended while driving in Washington, D.C. She woke up early the following Monday morning with the worst headache of her life, yet she continued into work. At work, the lawyers she worked with suggested she should see a doctor. She refers to this as her first clue she had a brain injury, as it hadn't even occurred to her to see a doctor until that point.

She recalls the doctor telling her she had whiplash, and she should take it easy. After a week at work, when she couldn't add up the hours on her timesheet, Anne was politely told to go home and rest.

A few weeks later, over the July Fourth weekend, she noticed that she had trouble tracking the fireworks display with her eyes, and realized she needed to seek help. She eventually saw a neurologist, who told her she had received a mild traumatic brain injury (mTBI). Anne was treated for headaches and the doctor ordered a range of tests, but he did not refer her to cognitive rehabilitation therapy.

She would eventually find a neuro-optometrist who helped her to understand she was having trouble reading because she was overdoing things, and thus needed to reduce activity until her eye-brain connection improved. The doctor gave her some basic eye-tracking exercises, and she began vision therapy class. She continued to work with him as well as with her other doctors to find therapies to help her keep getting better.

In 1999, Anne followed her then-boyfriend (now husband) to Austin, Texas, where she found a neurologist who was willing to take her on as a patient. He referred her to St. David's Rehabilitation Hospital, even though it had been more than two years since her brain injury. She had previously been told the brain can't recover beyond that point. She began getting rehab and started volunteering at the University of Texas. Anne and her boyfriend were married in October 2001, and they considered the wedding to be a rehabilitation exercise as it took a lot of project-management skills.

In March 2002, Anne and her husband moved back to Washington, D.C., where she eventually attended a Brain Injury Association conference and discovered the Northern Virginia Brain Injury Services (BIS). Anne was assigned a mentor through BIS, and she confided in him that she had hoped she had left her brain injury back in

Texas. BIS asked her to join the speakers' bureau, and she began speaking to groups about her brain injury.

At one event, Anne recalls attendees assuming she was one of the organizers because she didn't exhibit outward signs of a brain injury. At this time, few members of the public understood that a concussion is a brain injury. Anne was able to help shed light on the subject through her speaking engagements.

Anne also volunteered at the BIAA office. In March 2007, she was profiled in a *Washingtonian* magazine story, "I Wanted My Brain Back," which is available for download from the Mild TBI page in the Living with Brain Injury section of BIAA's website. She worked with BIAA staff and long-time advocate Robert DeMichelis on several policy issues, but especially the Annual Brain Injury Awareness Day on Capitol Hill. Anne was invited to speak on the briefing panel, "The Value of Rehabilitation," in March 2011. Shortly afterward, Anne and her husband moved back to Austin, where they reside today with their 8-year-old son, Daniel. Anne continues to serve on BIAA's Brain Injury Advisory Council as chairperson.

When asked how the BIAA has changed her life, Anne said: "I feel so blessed to be a part of this group. So many members are doing exciting things and have modeled for me where I want to go with my life and advocacy work. My first goal is to keep getting better and better, and watch other brain injury survivors solve problems and see their strengths. It has been amazing for me, so inspiring. I feel like we're thriving as a group. It's a lonely journey, especially if you don't get the proper care right away. It's been a blessing to have so many brothers and sisters taking this journey with me and pointing out different ways of doing things. It's so meaningful, and the inspiration I get from the other members is tremendous. We have an understanding of each other and have each other's backs."

This article originally appeared in Vol. 11, Issue 1 of THE Challenge!, the quarterly newsmagazine of the Brain Injury Association of America.

Sarah Lefferts

It started out like an ordinary September day for Sarah Lefferts in 2012. As she was walking, she suddenly slipped on wet tile flooring and fell backward, hitting her head on the floor. When she got up she was upset because she had spilled coffee on her dress, but she had no idea how much her life had changed in that split second.

Over the next several days, her concussion symptoms would progress. At the time of her fall, she was working full-time, also attending graduate school, and as a 20-something, she had an active social life. She was not okay with her new normal, and was frustrated that the healing wasn't more immediate. She wanted to get back to work and school, and wanted to push her recovery as quickly as she could.

Sarah, like most of us, didn't understand the recovery that was ahead of her, and neither did anyone around her. She said, "I learned a lot about how it was okay to be broken, and how I needed to communicate that to the people around me so they could understand enough to support me—even when I didn't understand my injury."

Her friends and family would go along to her doctor appointments and take notes so she could look back later to remember what they had talked about. Early in her recovery, she used a small notebook so she could keep her thoughts organized. She made to-do lists for everything, even basic stuff like showering and making food.

Sarah remembers going to the grocery store, and how she would freeze up as soon as she walked in. It was simply too much for her. All of the options to choose from, and she couldn't focus on what she was there to buy. She learned to make detailed lists, and also to save up her energy on days she had to go because she knew she would be completely exhausted afterward. So many people take this simple task for granted; yet for someone dealing with a brain injury, it is an overwhelming chore to tackle.

Her job was based on an ability to communicate and work with others. After her injury, she wasn't able to sustain conversations or be in groups. She didn't even have the energy to engage with other people, and having one long conversation would wipe her out.

Sarah felt that her identity had been taken away from her—everything that someone would have described her as, was now gone. It took her a long time to show excitement again, and she now appreciates the ability to show joyful emotions so much more than she had before.

"One of the hardest parts of the recovery wasn't the physical healing, but the social support. It's a real challenge to figure out how to communicate to your network about what's wrong and what you need from them. You look fine; you can walk and talk, so it's harder for them to understand what you're going through and what you need. Yet, it's critical that you seek support from them," commented Sarah.

Under her neurologist's care, Sarah returned to work on a partial schedule after her injury, gradually working her way back to full time within the first year. In 2014 she went back to grad school, taking one class at a time, with some academic flexibility to accommodate her slower speed in processing information. She went on to complete a triathlon in 2015 and graduated with her MA in May 2016.

Sarah wants others with a concussion to understand they're not alone—*and people do heal from this.* There are resources and a community out there to help you through it. It's challenging to advocate for yourself the way you must when that part of your brain has been damaged, but you need to put your own physical and mental health first, which is not something society teaches us.

When asked how the BIAA has changed her life, Sarah said: "The group of people I have met through the BIAA is empowering and supportive. BIAA taught me I am not alone in brain injury, and every injury is different. It blew me away when I realized how many people suffer from concussions and other brain injury. I feel like my responsibility on the other side of this injury is to help other people understand *this injury is often invisible, but you are not*—and it's okay to always keep striving to heal."

This article originally appeared in Vol. 11, Issue 2 of THE Challenge!, the quarterly newsmagazine of the Brain Injury Association of America.

Paul Bosworth

While living in Washington, D.C. and working for a leading computer manufacturer, Paul Bosworth received a TBI after he choked on chicken-fried rice. Alone in his kitchen, he passed out, hitting his head on the floor. When he came to, he still had food lodged in his throat, so he went into the bathroom in an attempt to remove it, causing tears in his throat. He then called his girlfriend to take him to the ER.

At first, the doctors were most concerned about the tears and bleeding. He was sent home, but was told he had suffered a concussion. He went back to work, but as the days went on, it became apparent he had suffered more brain damage than originally thought. He was having a hard time speaking, and would stutter frequently, and he was plagued with debilitating headaches. He had a difficult time reading and comprehending things. He eventually went to a neurologist whom ironically he met at a happy hour, who told him he had post-concussion syndrome (PCS).

After a conversation with fellow brain injury survivor, Anne Forrest, Paul decided to join the Brain Injury Advisory Council in 2009. He stated, "Finally, I could use my skills learned at my job to lend a hand post-mTBI."

In 2008, Paul began to realize he wasn't going to be able to continue working and went on long-term disability. He moved back home to south Louisiana to be near friends and family. Friends from his corporate life had been slowly and gradually leaving him—as they simply didn't understand that now he was living with the effects of this silent epidemic.

Back home, he began a support group called AMAZE. "AMAZE provides a space for caregivers and survivors to take a breath, and know they are not alone. Guest speakers visit our group's monthly meetings to share therapies or activities that add life every time. AMAZE is a place where a member will be understood, and not judged," said Paul. Thanks to doctor referrals, AMAZE has grown over the past seven years.

After a few years, he knew he needed to do something more to raise awareness, as well as occupy his time. He put together the first BBQ4TBI event, having a community barbeque in conjunction with a Jeep ride, and it was wildly successful. After doing it two years, the city of Breaux Bridge became involved, and it evolved into a bigger and more exciting event. Organizing the BBQ gave Paul a sense of belonging, and it became his "work" as he is still on long-term disability. It also challenges his brain, and allows him to relearn skills he had lost.

When asked how the BIAA has changed his life, Paul said, "BIAA provides me a unique platform so I am able to connect and learn more about what is being done to positively influence brain injury on several different levels.

I am also able to get a sense of what's coming down the pipe to help survivors and caregivers. Each March while I am in Washington, D.C. attending Brain Injury Awareness Day, I take a stand by showing up in my state lawmakers' office to effectively highlight brain injury from a first-person perspective."

"BIAA enables me to gain access to the people with the latest information and statistics, help those who are presenting research findings in public forums, as well as what Americans, both civilian and military alike, are doing to move the ball forward at the Brain Injury Awareness Day Fair. After all, we are together in this fight for better brain health."

This article originally appeared in Vol. 11, Issue 3 of THE Challenge!, the quarterly newsmagazine of the Brain Injury Association of America.

Stephanie Freeman

When she was only 14-years-old, Stephanie Freeman was involved in a rollover car crash, flipping five times on a country road. She sustained lung and brain damage as well as a shattered pelvis and other physical injuries. Stephanie spent two months in a coma at Palmyra Park Hospital in Albany, Georgia, and would go on to spend a total of four months and eight days in the hospital.

After being released from the hospital, she spent another six months completing rehabilitation before she was allowed to go back to school. Now a year behind her classmates, Stephanie went to summer school to catch up.

She graduated with the class of '96 and took a year off before attending Georgia Southwestern State University. She later graduated from Wiregrass Technical College with a degree in business.

In 2003, Stephanie began running in order to combat depression and anxiety. She's a strong believer in physical activity, and became committed to running and working out on a daily basis. She ran her first marathon in 2006, and has since run 10 marathons as well as numerous half marathons and 5Ks.

On July 10, 2006, Stephanie gave birth to her son, Range. She considers him to be her miracle baby, as she had been told after her accident she would never be able to conceive a child.

In 2013, Stephanie was working at the Boston Marathon at mile marker 25.5 when the Boston Marathon Bombing occurred. This event triggered Post-Traumatic Stress Disorder (PTSD) and brought up unresolved emotional trauma she had not dealt with as a teenager after her car accident. This event prompted her to start her foundation, Share Your Strong.

It took more than two years to establish the foundation, and she now uses it as a way to bring health, help, and inspiration to people who are going through brain trauma. She raises money through the marathons she runs and has even competed in fitness competitions to show that mental health can be combated without drugs.

One year after the bombing, Stephanie ran the Boston Marathon—as a way to come full circle with all she had been through in her life. Stephanie attended Brain Injury Awareness Day in March 2015 and was invited to join the Brain Injury Association of America Advisory Council shortly afterward.

She is currently furthering her education in natural healing reflexology and neuromuscular massage therapy in order to help others promote natural healing of the brain. Stephanie is also a certified trainer and mentor to high school students who want to improve their health; she helps them with their eating and exercise plans and encourages brain-healthy foods.

Her motto in life is "Never, ever give up!"

When asked how BIAA has changed her life, Stephanie said: "Being part of something that completely changed my life allows me to help others with the same problems I have faced. It touches my heart, and I am living with purpose by being part of this."

This article originally appeared in Vol. 11, Issue 4 of THE Challenge!, the quarterly newsmagazine of the Brain Injury Association of America.

Carole Starr

Carole Starr is now a published author, keynote speaker and the leader of the award-winning survivor group Brain Injury Voices. However, 18 years ago she was a teacher early in her career and an amateur violinist and singer who loved performing. On July 6, 1999, her car was broadsided in an accident—and she was completely unprepared for the way her life and self would change.

When she tried to go back to her regular activities six to eight weeks later, it became apparent more was wrong than just whiplash. It was only then that doctors told Carole she had suffered a traumatic brain injury (TBI).

She couldn't understand her extreme mental fatigue, heightened sensitivity to light and sound, and difficulty managing everyday tasks. She had to quit playing music because she couldn't tolerate the sound, and would have to rest for days after struggling to teach for only two hours. She was frustrated that she couldn't simply push through it.

As she began rehab, she started to understand more about TBI and why everything was so challenging for her. At the time, she believed she would make a full recovery.

Carole tried repeatedly to return to teaching and music, but each time she failed. It took her about eight years to accept her injury, and to acknowledge she wasn't going to get her old life back. She mourned the loss of her old life and her old self. Eventually, she began to embrace the new person she had become, and to focus on building a new life. Finding meaning in her experience, and paying it forward, were very important to her.

Carole said, "I didn't think I could ever come to terms with this new Carole, but eventually I did. I want to help others on this journey because it is *so* hard. I want to give others hope, to know that it *is* possible to have a happy, meaningful, productive life, even when coping with a disability. You have to let go of *what was* in order to live *what is*."

In 2010, Carole teamed up with her mentor, Bev Bryant, to found Brain Injury Voices, a survivor volunteer group in her home state of Maine. Their mission is simple: Educate, Advocate, Support. Their motto is all about paying it forward for others on the brain injury path.

In the past seven years, members of Brain Injury Voices have volunteered more than 15,000 hours, given more than 150 presentations, and mentored over 1,500 peers. Also, this year they were able to fundraise enough money to help some of their members, including Carole, to attend Congressional Brain Injury Awareness Day in Washington, D.C. on March 20, 2018.

It's only been in the last few years that Carole has been able to travel again, with support from friends and family. She now gives inspirational keynotes at brain injury conferences. "My goal is to travel the country as a brain injury speaker and to share what I've learned from my 18-year journey to help others," she says.

Carole's latest way to pay it forward is through her book, *To Root & To Rise: Accepting Brain Injury*, which was published in 2017. *To Root & To Rise* is a workbook intertwined with her memoir. Each chapter is about a different aspect of the grieving and acceptance process. It's designed in such a way that readers can choose which chapters to read, and they don't have to read them in order. Carole's teaching roots come out in this book. Each chapter includes questions and space for self-reflection, so readers can apply Carole's strategies to their own experience.

Through her book, keynotes and leadership of Brain Injury Voices, Carole is paying it forward and making a difference in the brain injury community.

Carole joined the BIAC shortly after attending her first Brain Injury Awareness Day in March of 2016.

When asked how the BIAA has changed her life, Carole replied, "I didn't have a passion for a cause before my injury, and now I do. For that, I am very grateful. BIAA helps me to focus on that passion. I like knowing there is a larger organization out there working for survivors, that we are not alone. I have the opportunity to become more involved and be a voice nationally. Doing that alongside BIAA means a lot to me."

This article originally appeared in Vol. 12, Issue 1 of THE Challenge!, the quarterly newsmagazine of the Brain Injury Association of America.

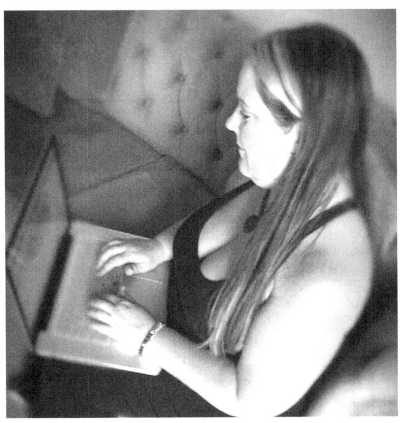

Advocacy work has become my passion,
mission, and career.

Chapter Twenty-Three

An Open Letter to Arianna Huffington

Dearest Arianna,

Three years ago, you gave me an opportunity. I was broken and alone—literally. I had suffered a traumatic brain injury from a fall on the ice, and had turned to writing as my therapy.

You gave me an outlet to share my voice—an advocacy platform—and thousands of fellow brain-injured folks from around the world listened.

As you held my hand during the initial phase of setting up my contributor site, you were kind, gentle, and encouraging.

I thanked you profusely for the opportunity, and each time you would take time to write back, *thanking me for the thank you.*

I looked up to you, as a beautiful, strong, confident woman who was paving the way in an online world of news media, allowing contributors to help you grow your readership while giving them a place to share their personal messages.

You appreciated those who were part of your virtual team. It was even rumored you were spotted reading MY book while waiting at your eye doctor's office in Beverly

Hills. Whether this is true or not, I believe you were proud of me for publishing a book from my collection of *Huffington Post* essays.

Because of YOU...I now have a thriving TBI Tribe on Facebook with over 8,000 survivors and caregivers from around the world.

Because of YOU...I have helped save lives—literally.

Because of YOU...hundreds of thousands of brain-injured people around the globe are feeling *a tiny bit less alone tonight.*

I was thrilled for you when you left *Huffington Post* to start *Thrive Global*. You have also graciously given me a platform to contribute there as well. It was a well-deserved move for you, and I applaud you for following your heart.

You are a remarkable woman, and I feel compelled to tell you so, as I am still a bit shell-shocked learning that *HuffPost* will no longer have 100,000 contributors helping them pave the way with revolutionary thinkers.

But it's all okay. I know my advocacy work will continue through other outlets (such as *Thrive*). We women know how to make the most of a situation, don't we?

From the very bottom of my heart, thank you dear Arianna, for being there for me when I needed you most!

Sincerely,

Resources

Here is a small list of resources, including the ones I have found helpful in my recovery, plus the ones I created. I hope they steer you in the right direction.

Brain Injury Association of America
www.biausa.org

United States Brain Injury Alliance
www.usbia.org

Brain Line
www.brainline.org

CTE Hope
www.cte-hope.org

Brain Injury Radio
www.blogtalkradio.com/braininjuryradio

Facebook — Amy's TBI Tribe
www.facebook.com/groups/792052120888627/

Faces of TBI (podcast, doctors resource guide, and suggested reading list)
www.facesoftbi.com

My doctors, clinics, and other resources in Minnesota:

Dr. Jeremy Schmoe, DC DACNB
Minnesota Functional Neurology
www.mnfunctionalneurology.com

Drs. Erin and Elizabeth, DC
Twin Life Chiropractic
www.twinlifechiropractic.com

Greg Santema, PT
Cranial Sacral Therapy
www.novacare.com

James Heuer, attorney
Heuer Fisher, P.A.
www.HeuerFischer.com

The Brain Injury Research Lab
www.samadanilab.com

About the Author

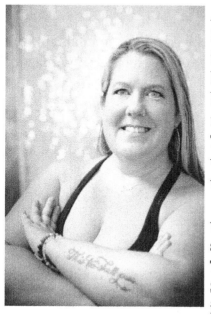

Amy sustained her TBI in February of 2014 after falling on a patch of ice and landing full-force on the back of her skull. She is still recovering, and advocating TBI awareness while traveling around the country with her Yorkie, Pixxie.

Amy is an award-winning author, keynote speaker, podcast host, and TBI advocate located in Saint Paul, Minnesota. She is a frequent contributor to *HuffPost, Good Men Project, Medium, The Mighty,* and *Thrive.* Her work has also been featured in *Yoga Today* and *Wagazine,* and she writes a column in *The Challenge!,* the Brain Injury Association of America's quarterly magazine.

She is a member of the Brain Injury Association of America's Advisory Council, and a volunteer for the Minnesota Brain Injury Alliance's Citizen's Advocates.

Passionate about sharing her story, Amy creates more awareness around this invisible injury that affects over 2.8 million Americans each year. She wants to bring an awareness and understanding to the world, and hopes people will have more compassion for those who look seemingly fine, *like she does*, but inside are struggling with memory or cognitive issues.

Her first two books received silver medals in the Midwest Book Awards and may be purchased on Amazon:

- *Life With a Traumatic Brain Injury: Finding the Road Back to Normal*
- *Surviving Brain Injury: Stories of Strength and Inspiration*

Amy is available for speaking at conferences and events, and may be reached by email: AmyZellmerTBI@gmail.com or via her website, www.facesoftbi.com

Made in the USA
Monee, IL
04 February 2020